BAMM CLINICAL DIRECTORS' SERIES

Clinical Director of Pathology
Tackling the role

Edited by
MICHAEL GALLOWAY

Foreword by
SUZANNE CHAPMAN

Series Foreword by
PETER LEES AND JENNY SIMPSON

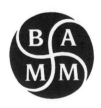

RADCLIFFE MEDICAL PRESS

© 1999 Michael Galloway

Radcliffe Medical Press Ltd
18 Marcham Road, Abingdon, Oxon OX14 1AA

British Library Cataloguing in Publication Data

A catalogue record for this book is available from the British Library.

ISBN 1 85775 343 7

Contents

Series Foreword

Managing the clinical service is a challenging occupation in which the role of the doctor has increased exponentially since the radical changes of the Thatcher government in the middle to late 1980s (is it really that long ago!). The involvement of clinicians in management was, of course, a fundamental tenet of the late Sir Roy Griffiths' advice in his response to the confidential enquiry into the NHS in 1983.

It is tempting to think that the challenges facing doctor managers have also increased dramatically but that would be to forget the context of the earlier times and the enormous culture change that has been achieved. Nevertheless, the complexity of the agenda that faces today's doctor managers, indeed all managers, has changed beyond all recognition.

Devolved management structures are the norm rather than an optional extra and the directorate model – in one form or another – is widely accepted as fundamental to effective trust management. It is here that the political and managerial is translated into practical action – no mean feat in this era of change mania and run-away demand inflation. The individuals who have taken the risk of leading directorates have seen a major change in their roles, from the early days of budget holders (or rather overspend blame-takers) to the current and developing roles as strategic clinical leaders, key to the future direction of their organisation. They have also experienced, however, the isolation of a 'different' career path, the status of clinical director and the unpopular management decision.

These individuals need help and a network of peers. They need a 'home' in which they can share their learning, share their successes, share their failures. BAMM does that – it is why the organisation exists and this series is a further building block in the framework of support for clinical directors. What is innovative about this series is its focus. The suggestion that specialty training in medicine is interchangeable would be met these days with some considerable scorn – registrars no longer hop across major specialty divides because it is too difficult. Focused training is the norm. Yet the clinician in management makes do with generic management texts which, excellent as they may be, do not recognise the enormous diversity of today's NHS. Managing a pathology service is just not the same as managing a cardiac surgery service.

This series is not about fostering differences but is about providing help with the context and practicalities of managing directorates – discrete and highly complex integral parts of the even more complex whole that is today's NHS hospital. It is the aim that along with standard texts clinician managers will have this, their directorate-specific text to help and thereby also achieve one of the fundamental aims of clinical governance – the sharing of learning, good ideas and best practice.

Peter Lees
Jenny Simpson
BAMM
April 1999

Foreword

Change, change and more change: the clinical director has a pivotal role which includes leading and developing strategic change for the directorate, but taking on the title does not come with a 'user manual'. Clinicians in disciplines such as pathology need to know about financial management, quality assurance, purchasing equipment, and 'health & safety' but we do not always get to grips with these until taking on a management role. Here is a 'shortcut' guide for clinical directors – the chapters on these important topics should be compulsory reading for anyone tackling the role.

The clinical director, essentially, learns 'on the job'. At times the role can seem a lonely one – 'on the one hand explaining and justifying management to clinical colleagues and on the other impressing on managerial colleagues the reality of clinical practice'. More than anything, the clinical director learns and benefits from networking and comparing notes with colleagues in similar positions. Many of the challenges and problems in pathology are not unique. What better than to learn from colleagues, either on a similar learning curve or those more experienced, who understand the problems and have 'been there, done that, got the T-shirt'.

At BAMM Pathology Network Group meetings the same issues were common to many, whether in a large teaching hospital or a small DGH. Some clinical directors had already dealt with complex change projects, such as changes to the 'on call' service or laboratory mergers. We realised there was much to learn from their experiences. Sharing these and the different solutions arrived at, gave fresh insight and perspectives to important issues facing clinical directors of pathology and revitalised the approach to them. So this book, in a way, represents the metaphorical 'pooling of T-shirts'. It pulls together the threads of the topics discussed at BAMM Pathology Network Group meetings and condenses them into an excellent series of practical and valuable chapters, dealing with specific, relevant topics. These range from the 'Corporate role of pathology' and 'Clinical governance', through to 'Benchmarking laboratory performance' and 'Changing working patterns', making an apposite and readable guide for anyone with an interest in managing pathology services.

This book is also testimony to the enthusiasm and commitment of its editor, Michael Galloway, the first chairman of the BAMM Pathology Network Group and to all those who have contributed chapters. The group members too played a large part in shaping content of the meetings which formed a nucleus for this book.

Change continues and there is no 'arrival point'. The clinical director travels on a voyage of discovery and adaptation: now we see the introduction of clinical governance as a framework embracing the quality and efficiency of a service, tomorrow, no doubt, there will be other changes, other challenges. Yet the same skills, awareness and background knowledge will be needed to tackle the role. A wealth of essential and practical information for clinical directors in pathology can be found here – topical and forward looking. It is reassuring to have such a useful guidebook for the journey!

Suzanne Chapman
Consultant Medical Microbiologist
Clinical Director, Rapid Diagnosis & Assessment
April 1999

Preface

This is the first in a series of books to be written by members of the British Association of Medical Managers (BAMM). It is hoped that this series of practical books will help clinical directors tackle their role as medical managers. This book has evolved from the meetings of the BAMM Pathology Network Group. The group held its first meeting in November 1994 and was attended by 20 clinical directors of pathology. It was clear that each clinical director brought a number of experiences and developments which could be shared usefully with all members of the group. As a result a number of workshops were organised over the following three years. The workshops were organised by one of the BAMM pathologists. Each workshop addressed one of the key areas of pathology management and these workshops therefore formed the basis of this book.

The book is aimed at consultants considering taking up the role of clinical director and we also hope it will be useful to those who are actually doing the job. In addition it may be a useful induction to pathology for laboratory business managers, especially if they have a general management background. When preparing this book it was not our intention to write another definitive management text. Instead, the aim of this book is to recount practical experiences from the BAMM Pathology Network Group. Throughout the book guidance to further reading is given and this includes reference to standard management text books.

In conclusion it is hoped that this book will help clinical directors achieve organisational development with the aim of improving the quality of their pathology service. The practical lessons that have been learnt from the BAMM Pathology Network Group deserve a wider audience. From a personal point of view it has been an exciting four years in which to be involved with such an enthusiastic group of medical managers who have participated in the BAMM Pathology Network Group meetings. Finally I would like to acknowledge the contribution of Tim Scott, who first suggested the idea of the book, and to thank Susan Nicholson who skilfully helped to prepare the manuscript.

Michael Galloway
April 1999

List of contributors

Helen Atkinson Research Assistant, Clinical Management Unit, Centre for Health Planning and Management, Keele University.

Judith Behrens Member of the Clinical Audit in Pathology Committee, Royal College of Pathologists, Clinical Director of Pathology and Consultant Haematologist, St Helier Hospital NHS Trust.

Andrew Boon Head of Cytopathology and Consultant Pathologist, St James's University Hospital, Leeds.

Roger Dyson Professor and Director, Clinical Management Unit, Centre for Health Planning and Management, Keele University.

Elizabeth Gaminara Clinical Director of Pathology and Consultant Haematologist, St Albans and Hemel Hempstead NHS Trust.

Angela Galloway Consultant Microbiologist, Public Health Laboratory, Newcastle General Hospital, Newcastle-upon-Tyne.

Michael Galloway Consultant Haematologist and former Clinical Director of Pathology, Bishop Auckland General Hospital, South Durham Health Care NHS Trust and past Chairman of the British Association of Medical Managers Pathology Network Group.

Suzanne Hartell Buyer, Diagnostic and Medical Equipment – Pathology, NHS Supplies.

Ian Lauder Vice President, Royal College of Pathologists, Professor of Pathology, Leicester Royal Infirmary & University of Leicester, former Clinical Director, Leicestershire Pathology Service and Chairman of the British Association of Medical Managers Pathology Network Group.

Denise Potter General Manager, Bishop Auckland General Hospital, South Durham Health Care NHS Trust.

Tim Scott Senior Fellow, British Association of Medical Managers.

Janet Shirley Medical Director and Consultant Haematologist, King Edward VII Hospital, Midhurst, West Sussex and Director, British Association of Medical Managers.

Shanthi Thomas Deputy Medical Director, Clinical Director of Pathology and Consultant Chemical Pathologist, Princess Alexandra Hospital, Harlow.

Barrie Woodcock Clinical Director of Pathology and Consultant Haematologist, Southport District General Hospital, Southport and Formby NHS Trust.

Introduction

DENISE POTTER
MICHAEL GALLOWAY

This book has been written at a time of considerable organisational change both within the NHS and within pathology. The introduction of the concept of clinical governance has focused attention on the quality of healthcare and not just the costs. Unfortunately there have been a number of well-publicised failings in pathology laboratories in which a poor-quality service has adversely affected patient care. As a result it will become increasingly important for clinical directors of pathology to be aware not only of the cost-effectiveness but also the quality of their service.

Clinical director of pathology – a pathologist's view

A number of factors which are important to the success of any quality improvement initiative have been identified.[1] The major components include clarifying roles and responsibilities; the development of appropriate data, including performance indicators that can be used to monitor and improve the quality of the service; appropriate incentives; and the development of teamwork. There is evidence that working in teams can have a beneficial effect on financial performance, quality of care and staff motivation.[2] Within pathology, teamwork is becoming increasingly complex as a result of initiatives such as multidisciplinary working and revised management structures, usually as a result of incorporating pathology into a larger directorate. It is therefore essential that the clinical director of pathology takes a lead in developing teamwork within the laboratory so that the concepts of clinical governance can be implemented. It is equally important that the managerial role of the consultant in each speciality is clearly defined and that they are supported in developing the role of a multidisciplinary team within the laboratory. These changes require leadership, a skill clinical directors of pathology will need to acquire.[1]

At trust level, pathologists will be key individuals in implementing clinical governance. This is a result of the wide remit pathologists have, not only within the clinical areas of a trust but also, particularly for microbiologists, in the non-clinical areas in relation to infection control. There is potential risk associated with this wide role of pathologists. This risk is best described as pathologists having the benefit of hindsight. For example, histopathologists performing postmortems may identify the reasons why things have gone wrong. Lessons and new ways of working should be learnt from this rather than using clinical governance as part of a disciplinary process or a way of settling old scores!

Clinical director of pathology – a general manager's view

In all but very rare cases, clinical directors are themselves clinicians. The dichotomy which may be neatly packaged within terms of an allocated number of sessions for clinical work and a further number for managerial work ignores the inherent difficulty in being a part-time worker and a part-time leader. In reality this dichotomy is generally played out in the modification of the clinical director (leader) role. The temporary nature of the clinical director role creates a longer-term vision of 'colleagues' not employees. The significance of the influence of longer-term team working amongst consultants should not be ignored, particularly as it is likely that some 30 years of working life may be spent at the same place with the same colleagues. Being an equal but temporarily in charge modifies the actions of even the most gung-ho clinical director, at least within their own speciality.

The appointment of clinical directors is also usually subject to approval by their consultant colleagues. This process in itself is likely to produce the appointment of the 'most accepted'. This further reinforces the team working element of the role. It is unlikely that the 'most accepted' would be the consultant whom the others felt would initiate wholesale reorganisation of departments or indeed challenge their individual performance. Whilst this reflects the reality of the job, i.e. autonomous professional interests versus the corporate management agenda, the difficulties of incorporating these interests cannot be underestimated. This skill of a clinical director has been described as being able to 'hunt with the service providers', as well as being able to 'run with the unit managers'.[3]

Clinical directorships for the future look rather more prescriptive. The role of clinical governance in trusts, performance frameworks and national service frameworks all serve to reinforce the more prescriptive nature of healthcare in the future. Clinical directors will be charged with the delivery of this 'prescription'. It will be interesting to review how comfortable a profession that arguably wants to 'play a bigger part in managing the health service, to protect their clinical freedom'[4] is when it finds itself leading the delivery of services which will reduce the opportunities for clinical freedom. A new agenda, more prescriptive, more limiting and explicitly tackling priorities and rationing from both national and local perspectives is outlined in *A First Class Service: quality in the new NHS*.[5] This time the government's aim is to review performance, individual and corporate, in a way that is clinically meaningful to the staff.

It remains to be seen whether clinical directors seize this opportunity for management or whether the more prescriptive and 'managed' nature of healthcare and subsequently the professionals within it reduces the added value to trusts of clinicians participating. The balance of attempting to incorporate professionals into the management agenda appears theoretically easier now as the management agenda has actually become a management agenda for clinical change and excellence. Whether in fact a service benchmarked as acceptable will be pushed the extra mile by clinical directors who are used to incorporating colleagues' autonomous styles must be in doubt.

It seems in pulling together the clinical director model for management the trust must look at the way in which clinical directors are appointed, the expectations of the postholder, their tenure in post and the time commitment required to address the agenda. Perhaps for the first time managers within directorates supporting clinical directors will be working to deliver the same priorities as their clinical colleagues. It may be the end of the clinical director model of management being used as a management vehicle of control, 'the incorporation of professionals themselves into managerial roles, subject to managerial parameters'.[6]

Pulling it all together within an organisation relies heavily on development of strategies jointly with relevant services. Activity within pathology has a knock-on effect for the financial control of the laboratory services. The development of budgets to support service level agreements is beneficial in identifying increased activity and its associated cost. However, clinical directors must be cautious of the supposed wisdom that service level agreements bring costs under control. This may be true within elective specialities where demand can be controlled, however, the devolvement of a budget to an emergency speciality with no capacity to stem demand may only be shifting the overspend around the organisation. This has been particularly true in terms of acute medicine over recent years, which nationally has seen huge increases in workload. Whilst financial support has been available this has largely been to address specific projects in terms of managing winter pressures – the principle that emergency beds must always be available.

Once again the new NHS agenda will require areas such as pathology to develop services, not in consultation with other specialities but rather at a subspeciality or even disease-based level. Examples of this have already been evidenced with pathology departments responding to the Calman–Hine initiatives for cancer service development.[7] Agreements for reporting frameworks and turnaround times for tests should have been reached for each cancer type. This requires the pathology department to be both flexible in its approach to activity management and to adapt to the prescriptive nature of other specialities' clinical service reviews.

Perhaps, therefore, service level agreements are to become a misnomer being replaced with service delivery agreements.

Finally, whilst recognising all the limitations of vested interests, professional autonomy and demand-led service delivery, some model of clinical management must pull it all together. Of course the new NHS agenda is precisely about pulling it all together from a patient's perspective. The boundaries of departments, trusts, primary and secondary care are nonsensical when from a patient's perspective it is just stages and management of the same disease. From a clinical director's position the challenges are all about creating a desire amongst staff to change as a result of benchmarking and to balance the ideology of an improved clinical service for patients which may actually not improve the lot of those providing the service. The bridge to fill the implementation gap between 'what should be' and 'what is' is now a centrally controlled requirement.

Conclusion

There have been many centrally led initiatives over the years which it was anticipated would offer the golden goal in terms of clinical management of services. Programmes such as the resource management initiative, GP fundholding and contracting were designed to improve information to clinicians, offering hope for improved management of resources and better clinical quality. Of course, in some areas, some of these aims were met. Clinical governance does give the clinician the opportunity to be directly involved in defining the quality of a service by development of guidelines, setting standards of care, etc.[8]

Decisions about service priorities and standards will inevitably become more transparent and offer the greatest opportunity for the clinical director to strengthen both the management and leadership elements of the job. However, there is no panacea for each individual project or management task. A series of plans must be in place – selling an ideal to staff without a supporting process achieves only frustration with one's existing lot, whereas implementing a process without selling the rationale becomes bureaucracy.

In order to both achieve and to monitor change in pathology the clinical director must first ensure that processes are in place. Such processes include human resource management, formal and informal communication networks. Information on activity, effectiveness and service delivery must dovetail with financial control processes. Furthermore the clinical director must be an experienced influencer of opinion – understanding that different messages will be required to sell the same package to all the varied professionals in the directorate who of course will maintain their own clinical and intellectual preferences even within a managed multidisciplinary service.

References

1 Koeck C (1998) Time for organisational development in health-care organisations. *BMJ*. **317**: 1267–8.

2 Firth-Cozens J (1998) Celebrating teamwork. *Qual Health Care*. **7**: S3–7.

3 Packwood T, Keen J and Buxton M (1992) Process and structure: resource management and the development of sub-unit organisational structure. *Health Services Management Research*. **5**: 66–76.

4 Smith R, Grabham A and Chantler C (1989) Doctors becoming managers. *BMJ*. **298**: 311.

5 Secretary of State for Health (1998) *A First Class Service: quality in the new NHS*. Department of Health, London.

6 Harrison S and Pollitt C (1994) *Controlling Health Professionals*. Open University Press, Birmingham.

7 Calman K and Hine D (1995) *A Policy Framework for Commissioning Cancer Services*. Department of Health, London.

8 Donaldson LJ and Gray JAM (1998) Clinical governance: a quality duty for health organisations. *Qual Health Care*. **7**: S37–44.

1

Clinical directorates: background

TIM SCOTT

Since the 1960s, a variety of commentators have been concerned about roles of doctors, nurses and other clinical professionals within the management of hospitals and, more generally, the NHS. Academics and others pointed to what they saw as a gulf between doctors and managers and a variety of initiatives over the years have had this as one focus of their concerns.

The elaborate arrangements within the Grey book (the 1974 re-organisation) for the Area Medical Advisory Committee (AMAC) as well as the cogwheel structure at hospital level are manifestations of this. But what these achieved was no more than advisory mechanisms for tapping into the clinical voice rather than any joint management mechanism. The experience of many managers and indeed of clinicians was that doctors and others had no involvement in the implementation of their advice but could 'shroud wave' and block change without taking responsibility for resolving financial and other pressures.

Functional management

At this point in time, management arrangements, and therefore budgets, bore little resemblance to the pattern we see in the late 1990s. Many budgets were still held at district level, for example physiotherapy and occupational therapy, and those budgets that were held at hospital level were held on a functional basis. That is, there was a nursing budget broken down perhaps into out-patients, accident and emergency (A&E), and wards. There would be a medical staff budget, often held by the personnel department, since most medical staff, at least in non-teaching hospitals, were paid at a regional level and had contracts with the regional health authority. The pharmacist would hold the hospital or even district-wide drugs budget and there would be budgets for porter-ing, medical records, catering, training and medical secretaries. The vast majority of these budgets would be held by administra-tors, who were accountable through an administrative hierarchy.

Griffiths's review

Sir Roy Griffiths's fundamental review of the management of the NHS (the first as he reminded us since the Bradbeer Report in 1954) saw this as a primary concern. In this report, framed as a letter to the Secretary of State, Griffiths suggested experiments in what he called 'management budgeting'. This was to be a form of responsibility accounting with budgets framed around doctors, or groups of doctors, who, in financial terms, he saw as the prime drivers of expenditure. 'It is the actions of doctors, working as leaders of clinical teams, that lead to expenditure of funds and budgets will provide a means by which they can accept responsi-bility' was his view.

The management budgeting experiments were driven at regional and local level, rather than having any national focus or leadership. In all number of hospitals they were seen as an attempt to control doctors and resulted in confrontation between the finance function and the medical profession. In fact they became increasingly unpopular and were seen as a source of friction by such bodies as the British Medical Association (BMA).

When Ian Mills, a senior partner from management consultants Price Waterhouse, was appointed to the NHS Executive as the NHS's first director of financial management, he saw the management budgeting programme as one of his key tasks. In late 1986, in Health Notice number 34, he launched the re-engineered and re-visioned programme to be known as resource management, which was to spring phoenix-like from the ashes of management budgeting.

Resource management

There is always an iteration between central policy and what goes on in the NHS. The NHS prefers to invent things itself and to draw from other health services and other health systems and always 'interprets' central policy within its own framework. Increasingly we have also seen central policy makers recognising this effect and outlining ends whilst being less specific about the means. Such was to be the case with the management arrangements and particularly management structures which were associated with the resource management programme. There was already interest in the NHS in one or two places in changing the local management arrangements to involve doctors and nurses more fully. Some of those locations saw the resource management programme as providing validation that they sought, as well as an opportunity to tap into, central funds. Guy's Hospital, in particular, had visited Johns Hopkins in the USA and determined that there were aspects of their way of working which they wished to try. For them, resource management offered an ideal opportunity. Other hospitals, including Southampton University Teaching Hospital, were also engaged with the Hopkins model but did not feature in the early parts of the resource management programme. The Griffiths legacy of individual general managers had meant that every hospital could determine its own local management arrangements within the broad principle of general management and some had borrowed, or even invented, ways of involving clinical staff more fully.

Management models

Although the NHS popular press (*Health Services Journal*, *Hospital Doctor*, *Nursing Times* and so on) had picked up items of interest around these newly emerging structures and arrangements, there had been little formal dissemination. The convening of a group in 1989 under the banner of the resource management programme provided an opportunity for debate and discussion and for some consolidation and written record. A two-day workshop was translated into a publication which appeared as an Institute of Health Services Management (IHSM) booklet entitled *Models of Clinical Management* in 1990. This booklet, the circulation of which was funded by the NHS Executive, set out some aspects of the existing models, focusing not only on the structures but also on the processes by which such models worked and the roles and responsibilities taken by different individuals. For many in the NHS this was their first exposure to the detail of the clinical directorate model.

This model was clearly associated with the resource management initiative. The symposium and publication had been funded by the resource management programme and for many in the NHS it became the central message of resource management. Whilst the NHS Executive continued to maintain its position that it was for individual hospitals to determine management arrangements and that there was no central fiat for clinical directorates, at a more local level this was often disregarded. Sir Donald Wilson, chairman of Mersey Regional Health Authority, was said to have told all the hospitals in the region to adopt the directorate structure and other, more subtle pressures emerged in other locations. One obvious result of this was to alert the professional bodies. The BMA in particular began receiving a variety of phone calls from members asking for advice and guidance and they, the Royal College of Nursing (RCN), the IHSM and others began producing leaflets and hand-outs designed to alert their members to the possibilities and potential problems inherent in the directorate model.

Founding of BAMM

The British Association of Medical Managers (BAMM) can trace its beginnings back to this period and particularly to the establishment of clinical directorates. In 1990 Dr Jenny Simpson, then working at Sheffield Children's Hospital, convened a meeting of clinical directors from a number of hospitals including, particularly, those in the resource management initiative. After discussion it became clear that the doctors in this group had similar problems, not least that there had been very little investment in their own development and education. With support from the Department of Health this group visited the American College of Physician Executives (ACPE) national conference. They found a well-established body of doctors engaged in management, with training development programmes and a supportive infrastructure. In their minds BAMM was borne and the initial constitution was written some four months later.

From the beginning, BAMM's mission was not only to support doctors who wanted to engage with the management of the NHS but to work with others on the broader agenda of the involvement of clinical staff in management. During the lengthy internal debates about BAMM's stance as a unidisciplinary organisation the message was often repeated, 'whilst we remain as a unidisciplinary organisation we must work closely with nurses and others to make clear that we believe in multidisciplinary working'.

The principles of clinical management

As clinical directorates spread throughout the NHS, the professional bodies continued to field enquiries from members as to their opportunities and concerns about such arrangements. As BAMM began to work collaboratively with the other professional bodies, the opportunity to take a single position and speak in a united way on these matters emerged.

It was agreed that the professional bodies would work together to try to produce a single agreed statement of guidance for their respective members. Supported by the NHS Executive, a research project was undertaken with a substantial literature search, a number of site visits and the distribution of a questionnaire. This was deliberately targeted at what were perceived as leading sites and the intention was to determine the key principles for the involvement of clinical staff in management. The subsequent document proved very helpful to trusts busy rethinking their management arrangements in the light of the then escalating drive towards directorate structures.

The rapid pace of change in the field meant that there was considerable concern about the datedness of the guidance and within two years a follow-up project had been launched to look at the practical advice to provide to trusts on putting those principles into practice. Once again, the idea was to draw on the leading-edge trusts. This time each of the professional organisations involved (BAMM, BMA, IHSM and RCN) trawled their member-ship for trusts that the members considered to be 'excellent sites'. These lists were then brought together and the small area of overlap and consensus determined. Multidisciplinary site visits were arranged and a day was spent in each trust talking through with staff at every level their perceptions of whether the organisa-tion was genuine in its involvement of clinical staff, the stage that it had reached and the way in which it had achieved this.

This work was documented in two booklets, *Principles into Practice*[1] and a companion volume which contains a set of relevant documents from each of the exemplar sites. Different sites docu-mented their management arrangements in different ways but the companion volume provided job descriptions, descriptions of planning and budget setting processes, and guidance on the roles of key groups and key individuals. The intention was to allow the rest of the NHS to draw on this repository of material. The research suggested four key principles (Box 1.1) (extended from the three put forward from the original research) and nine imple-mentation tests (Box 1.2). It was suggested that individuals who were concerned about the organisation in which they found them-selves, should apply the nine implementation tests to see whether there was a real commitment by management to the involvement of clinical staff. It provided a simple self-assessment of the degree to which clinical management was a reality or a fiction.

Box 1.1: Four key principles

- Decentralised management: directorates or their equivalent with decision-making responsibility, devolved budgetary responsibility

- Flexible adaptive management arrangements, changing over time

- The multidisciplinary team as a core concept; the concerns of all professionals represented at trust management group level

- The development of shared views of clinical services between clinical staff in providers and purchasers

---

Box 1.2: Nine implementation tests

Directorates or their equivalent:

- in place

- tackling significant care issues

- involving all staff (communication)

- supported (staff and information)

- involved (structure)

- involved (process)

- committed to training and organisational development

- directorates, general practitioners (GPs) and purchaser staff in discussion and debate

- directorates managing income and expenditure within agreed business plan

---

The key is the creation of a single decision-making body for the organisation, bringing together the statutory board and the directorates. The diagram in Figure 1.1 shows the overlapping groups. What is crucial is that the central group brings together the accountability and governance systems within the organisation.

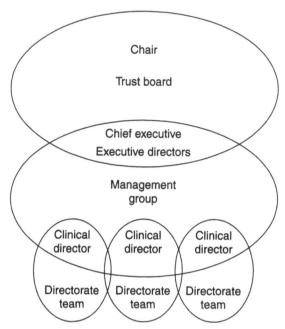

Figure 1.1 Trust management structure.

One problem observed in many trusts is where the opportunity exists to bypass such a single body. If the organisation allows and supports other routes to decisions, either through corridor politics or executive strategy groups or any such device, then great damage will be done to the devolved management arrangements. It is often easier, particularly for executive managers, to work on an individual basis with directorates or even with professionals within directorates. Such approaches, if not handled with extreme care, run the risk of undercutting the whole principle of directorates.

Within such a structure the clinical director becomes a pivotal role. The vast majority continue to work clinically and find themselves moving backwards and forwards between the world of clinical practice and the managerial world. They need expertise in both worlds and in particular the ability to translate from one world to another. They find themselves in the role of go-betweens: on the one hand explaining and justifying management to clinical colleagues and on the other impressing on managerial colleagues the reality of clinical practice. Whilst most clinical directors are doctors, there is no reason why this should be so. A small percentage has always been drawn from other professions and it is clear that any clinical professional can take on this role successfully. What is important is genuine knowledge and understanding of clinical process gained from experience, and continued close contact with the wide range of clinical professionals who deliver healthcare.

Clinical directors do not work alone. Most clinical directors have a business manager to support them and usually a manager to represent the largest group of staff within the directorate, be they nurses or technicians. Some large directorates have quite elaborate management arrangements with a number of subdirector management teams, whilst others will have a single management team. The typical directorate budget is around £5.3m but the range is very considerable; from less than £1m to more than £15m.[2]

Few clinical directors have any training or development prior to appointment. In some disciplines, particularly pathology and radiology, there had long been tradition of clinicians holding budgets. However, as the rest of this book makes clear, the role of the clinical director is considerably more than that of a budget holder and in particular the need to participate actively in organisational strategy and corporate decision-making meant that most appointees had development needs.

One common issue in trusts was the idea that clinical director posts were for a three-year period. This was, to some extent, a link back to advisory medical roles in a cogwheel structure since there was never any national guidance that determined such arrangements. In fact clinical directors have never been a part of any form of central guidance, constituting as they do local management arrangements. The result of this popular myth, however, was to see, in some trusts at least, a high turnover of clinical directors and the post becoming slightly token and 'Buggins turn'. Again research by BAMM suggests that clinical directors are in post for seven or eight years in a number of places and in fact this would seem to be an appropriate time in a complex and difficult job that requires a degree of experience to undertake well.

Summary

This chapter has endeavoured to provide a context and background to help readers understand the role of clinical director and directorate management. It has attempted to provide some sense of the history of the involvement of clinical staff in management, as well as give some indication of the approaches adopted. It makes clear the central role of clinical directors in such an approach and recognises the need to support such individuals. Clinical directors will increasingly find themselves at the very centre of clinical governance arrangements, for it is in clinical directorates where clinical service quality takes place. The ability to mediate between the managerial core of the organisation and the teams that deliver clinical care will be critical to both the maintenance and development of standards and the culture of continuous improvement.

Key point summary

- Clinical directorates with devolved decision making should be the basis for decentralised management arrangements.

- The key to devolved management is the creation of a single decision-making body bringing together the statutory board and the directorates.

- The organisation must not allow other routes for decision making to by-pass such a single body.

References

1 British Association of Medical Managers, British Medical Association, Institute of Health Services Management, Royal College of Nursing (1996) *Principles into Practice. The involvement of clinical staff in the management of NHS trusts.* BAMM, Stockport.

2 British Association of Medical Managers (1997) *Leading Clinical Services – the evolving role of the clinical director.* BAMM, Stockport.

2

Clinical governance

MICHAEL GALLOWAY

The new Labour Government has given a clear commitment to the development of the NHS.[1] The internal market has been abandoned and has been replaced by a framework that will facilitate co-operation and openness.[2] At the centre of the Government's aim to improve quality is the statutory duty of clinical governance.[3] In this chapter an outline of the concept of clinical governance is given and the implications for a clinical director of pathology is discussed.

Clinical governance

The definition of clinical governance is given in Box 2.1. The background to the development of clinical governance has been documented elsewhere[4,5] and involved concern around a number of areas including:

- Under the previous government's internal market too much emphasis had been placed on the costs of healthcare rather than the quality of the service.

- There were a number of serious clinical failures which had adverse effects on patient care.

- Previous quality improvement initiatives such as audit, research and development, and evidence-based practice remained fragmented within individual healthcare organisations.

Clinical governance has four dimensions that are shown in Box 2.2.[4] As can be seen, clinical governance embraces both the quality and efficiency of a service. Under new arrangements chief executives will be responsible for ensuring the quality of the services provided by their trust. The chief executive will also be expected to ensure that there are appropriate local arrangements in place so that the trust board has firm assurances that their responsibilities for quality are being met.

Box 2.1: What is clinical governance?

Clinical governance can be defined as a framework through which NHS organisations are accountable for continuously improving the quality of their services and safeguarding high standards of care by creating an environment in which excellence in clinical care will flourish.[3]

Box 2.2: Dimensions of clinical governance

- Professional performance
- Resource use
- Risk management
- Patients' satisfaction with the service provided

In many organisations this will be arranged through the creation of a subcommittee of the trust. It is likely that in many trusts a lead clinician will be appointed to develop clinical governance. One of the first tasks will be to pull together all of the separate initiatives that have been implemented in the NHS over recent years into one coherent organisational structure with the development of a clear strategy. The components that form the basis of clinical governance are shown in Box 2.3. It should not be assumed, however, that the implementation of clinical governance involves a series of organisational changes resulting in the establishment of clinical governance committees, etc. In order to place quality at the centre of a trust's activity, an organisational-wide transformation will be required.

Box 2.3: Components of clinical governance[1]

- Quality improvement processes are in place, e.g. clinical audit

- Development of clinical leadership skills

- Evidence-based practice is implemented

- Clinical risk reduction programmes are in place

- Adverse events are detected and lessons are learnt

- Patient complaints are addressed and lessons are learnt

- Poor clinical performance is identified and addressed

- The quality of data collected to monitor clinical care is of a high standard

- Programmes for continuing professional development are in place

---

Three interrelated areas in an organisation, i.e. culture, systems and structures will all have to be changed in order to facilitate the implementation of clinical governance.[2] In addition the development of clinical governance will also be facilitated by the establishment of multidisciplinary teams that will have the responsibility for implementing quality improvements.[6]

Clinical governance will sit at the centre of a trust's activity. There will be a number of external influences that will facilitate the development of clinical governance. This includes the establishment of the National Institute for Clinical Excellence and National Service Frameworks (Figure 2.1). These will provide evidence-based guidelines together with a framework for the delivery of a service. This approach will be familiar to those clinicians who have been involved in implementation of the Calman–Hine report.[7] These issues are further developed in Chapter 7. The performance of trusts, particularly in relation to the quality of a service, will be externally assessed by the Commission for Health Improvement and the development of a National Performance Framework. Underpinning these national initiatives is the duty of individual doctors to keep up to date, perform consistently well and to be an effective team player.[8, 9]

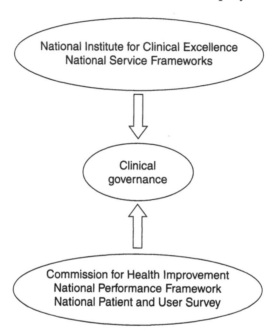

Figure 2.1 The framework for the implementation of clinical governance.[3] National Service Frameworks will set common standards for treatment. The National Institute for Clinical Excellence (NICE) will act as a nationwide appraisal body for new and existing treatments. The Commission for Health Improvement (CHI formerly known as CHIMP) will carry out reviews of trusts to ensure delivery of quality services. The National Framework for Assessing Performance will focus on the quality and efficiency of trusts. An annual national survey will provide feedback from patients and users.

The role of the clinical director of pathology

The clinical director of pathology will be the key individual for ensuring that clinical governance is implemented within his or her directorate. The starting point must be a clear job description reflecting the roles and responsibilities that will be required. These are outlined in Box 2.4. For any clinical director taking on this role this is a challenging agenda. Leadership skills will need to be developed by the clinical director. The clinical director should agree an appropriate level of remuneration for the job. For most directorates this will involve payment of two additional sessions.[10,11]

As the clinical director's job evolves with the implementation of clinical governance there will need to be some discussion regarding roles and responsibilities between the clinical director and the medical director. A suggested split between the roles of the medical director and clinical director in relation to the management of other consultants is shown in Box 2.5.

Box 2.4: Key elements that should be included in the job description of a clinical director of pathology (based on Ref. 10)

- Full management responsibility for all resources including financial, staff, equipment and facilities used by the directorate

- Develop a directorate strategy and ensure that it is aligned to the trust strategy

- To agree, implement and deliver the directorate annual business plan

- To ensure that effective management systems are in place to improve the quality and cost effectiveness of the service, e.g. clinical audit, adverse event reporting, patient complaints, risk management and benchmarking

- To ensure that all departments are accredited by Clinical Pathology Accreditation CPA (UK) Ltd

- To ensure that systems to improve clinical practice are in place, e.g. protocol development, pathways of care and evidence-based practice

- To ensure that training programmes are in place for all staff and consultants achieve the annual continuing medical education/continuing professional development scheme (CME/CPD) credits as defined by the Royal College of Pathologists

- To ensure that appraisal is performed for all staff

- To ensure that if poor performance is identified, it is addressed

- To develop multidisciplinary teams within the directorate at speciality level

---

Box 2.5: Clinical governance and the management of consultants – the role of the clinical director and medical director

Medical director role	Joint role	Clinical director role
• Disciplinary procedures	• Job plans	• Management performance
• Consultant contracts		– business plan
• Clinical performance – addressing areas of concern identified by a clinical director		– financial performance
		– quality of the service
		• Continuing medical education / continuing professional development
		• Study leave
		• Clinical performance – identifying any areas for concern
		• Ensuring that external peer review is undertaken, e.g. all departments are accredited by CPA (UK) Ltd

---

Conclusion

With the implementation of clinical governance, clinical directors of pathology are going to be the key individuals within the directorate. They will need to take the lead in developing the systems within their directorate that will ensure a quality service is delivered. Furthermore, they will have an important role in organisational change, particularly in relation to change in culture and team development. A checklist for the areas that clinical directors of pathology should be addressing is given in Box 2.6. The themes which have been developed in this chapter are explored in further detail throughout the rest of this book.

Box 2.6: Clinical governance – a checklist for clinical directors of pathology (adapted from Ref. 10)

System	Process established?	Process explicit within organisation?	Process amenable to monitoring?	Reporting arrangements?	Implementation of findings/lessons monitored?	Levers and sanctions in place to make it work?
Roles and responsibilities – job descriptions clearly outlining responsibilities must be in place for all staff (Chapter 4)						
Systems for external peer review are in place, e.g. all departments must be accredited by CPA (UK) Ltd						
Quality improvement process integrated into directorate quality programme. Is there a lead clinician for clinical audit in the directorate? (Chapter 7) Does the directorate have a quality manager? (Chapter 6)						
Evidence-based practice – Is there access to appropriate information sources, e.g. Cochrane Library, etc.?						
Clinical risk reduction: Are programmes in place and of high quality? Does the Infection Control Committee function well? (Chapter 3) Is there a Transfusion Committee? (Chapter 3) Does the directorate have a health and safety officer? (Chapter 12) Are near patient testing policies in place? (Chapter 3)						
Adverse events – detected and investigated and are lessons learnt and translated into change in practice?						
Systematic learning from clinical complaints with translation into change in practice						
Are programmes for continuing professional development and continuing medical education in place? Do all consultants achieve the appropriate number of CME/CPD credits?						
Quality of data for monitoring clinical care of consistently high standard, e.g. service level agreements with appropriate monitoring (Chapter 8) benchmarking cost-effectiveness (Chapter 10) benchmarking quality (Chapter 6)						
Are clinical leadership skills developed at the departmental level?						
Poor clinical performance identified early and dealt with with skill, speed and sensitivity to avoid harm to patient						

Key point summary

- Clinical governance is now a statutory duty for chief executives of trusts.

- Trust boards will want to ensure that procedures are in place to ensure that a quality service is provided by their organisation.

- Clinical directors of pathology will have key roles in implementing clinical governance within their directorate.

- The clinical director of pathology will need to ensure that he or she develops the appropriate skills to achieve organisational change that will be required to implement clinical governance.

References

1 Secretary of State for Health (1997) *The New NHS: modern, dependable*. HMSO, London.

2 Donaldson LJ and Gray JAM (1998) Clinical governance: a quality duty for health organisations. *Qual Health Care*. **7**: S37–44.

3 Secretary of State for Health (1998) *A First Class Service: quality in the new NHS*. Department of Health, London.

4 Scally G and Donaldson LJ (1998) Clinical governance and the drive for quality improvement in the new NHS in England. *BMJ*. **317**: 61–5.

5 Ayres PJ, Wright J and Donaldson LJ (1998) Achieving clinical effectiveness: the new world of clinical governance. *Clinician in Management*. **7**: 106–11.

6 Firth-Cozens J (1998) Celebrating teamwork. *Qual Health Care*. **7**: S3–7.

7 Calman K and Hine D (1995) *A Policy Framework for Commissioning Cancer Services*. Department of Health, London.

8 General Medical Council (1998) *Good Medical Practice*. GMC, London.

9   General Medical Council (1998) *Maintaining Good Medical Practice*. GMC, London.

10   British Association of Medical Managers (1998) *Clinical Governance in the New NHS*. BAMM, Stockport.

11   British Association of Medical Managers (1997) *Leading Clinical Services – the evolving role of the clinical director*. BAMM, Stockport.

3

Corporate role of pathology

ANGELA GALLOWAY
ANDREW BOON
SHANTHI THOMAS
MICHAEL GALLOWAY

Pathologists as a group are often regarded by many as 'the back-room boys', although increasingly other consultants and general practitioners do recognise the different disciplines within pathology. The general public now realise that a pathologist is not just someone who does postmortems. Pathologists are a mixed group of specialists who, unlike radiologists, cannot do each other's jobs. They all are likely to be members of the Royal College of Pathologists and many may also be members of the Royal College of Physicians.[1] Organisationally there will usually be a director of pathology, although the whole directorate may involve other specialities, e.g. radiology and pharmacy. In pathology a lead consultant will usually be nominated in each of the disciplines.[2] In addition, pathologists often share common accommodation, general office facilities, a general manager and have similar problems with regard to receipt, storage and disposal of specimens. Changes in the NHS have impacted substantially on the diagnostic services (Box 3.1).

An important corporate role of the pathologist is to provide strategic leadership in the planning and delivery of the services.[3] This should take into account the rapidly developing clinical role which is occurring in all the disciplines and the enormous technological developments that have been made in the processing aspects of the service. It is recognised that it is essential to provide not just a clinically effective but also a cost-effective service.

Box 3.1: Changes in the NHS – impact on pathology

- Decreased number of beds available

  ↓

- Decreased length of stay

  ↓

- Increase in emergency admissions

  ↓

- Increased need for investigations
- Increased access to investigations
- Rapid turnaround of results to assist decreased length of stay

---

Each consultant is involved in the pre-analytical, analytical and post-analytical stage of laboratory testing but the clinical role will vary with the discipline and to some extent on individual practice within the discipline (Box 3.2). An effective pathology service is of critical importance to the overall effectiveness of the trust and primary care.

Box 3.2: The three phases of laboratory work

- Pre-analytical
  - liaison with users
  - choice of tests (laboratory handbook)
  - design of request forms
  - transport arrangements

continued

- Analytical
  - choice of equipment
  - choice of method
  - regular review of methods
  - protocols for testing
  - reporting (histopathologist)
- Post-analytical
  - verification of reports
  - interpretation
  - clinical liaison
  - advise on further tests
  - monitoring demand

The operational role of pathology within the trust is to provide an efficient and safe service to meet patient needs. The various aspects of this role are illustrated in Figure 3.1.

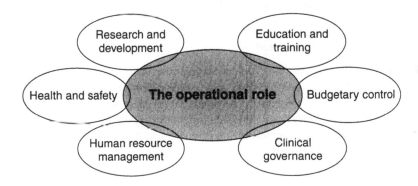

Figure 3.1 The operational role of pathology.

Clinical governance

NHS trusts' principal statutory duties have until now been financial, however, now every trust is required to embrace the concept of 'clinical governance' so that quality issues are addressed both at an organisational and at an individual level.[4] Processes which will assist in a quality organisation include:

- clinical audit

- evidence-based practice

- good internal and external communication

- risk management (Box 3.3)

- recognition and investigation of adverse events

- investigation of complaints

- assessment of performance

- continuous professional development

- information systems (collection and review of data).

All of these apply within pathology. The technical quality of the laboratory is assessed through internal and external quality assurance schemes and through laboratory accreditation – usually with CPA (UK) Ltd. Specific examples of aspects of clinical governance will be considered under each speciality.

Box 3.3: Risk management

Most trusts subscribe to the Clinical Negligence Scheme for Trusts (CNST). Meeting the standards set by CNST also ensures that clinical and organisational standards are in place. An example of the corporate role is in investigating (and rectifying) clinical teams not acting on critical test results. Through the untoward incident reporting system, these mistakes can be detected. Pathology should ensure that systems are in place so that clinical teams act on test results.

Health and safety

Health and safety is a statutory corporate duty of heads of departments and is considered separately in Chapter 12.

Human resource management

Staff are the most valuable resource and in pathology account for about 65% of the cost of the service. Human resource management constitutes an important aspect of the corporate role. This includes recruitment and retention of staff, training, development, monitoring sickness absence (Figure 3.2), appraisal and implementing effective communication processes.

Budgetary control

Pathology accounts for approximately 3% of a hospital's budget.[5] The number of requests and the range of diagnostic tests in pathology have been steadily rising. Within a cash-limited service, budgetary control is an important corporate role. It involves controlling demand with the use of guidelines, the effective use of supplies and regular reviewing of the staffing structures so as to reduce costs.[6] The use of multiskilled staff covering 24 hours a day, 365 days a year on a shift system has in some trusts resulted in reduced cost and improved quality.[7]

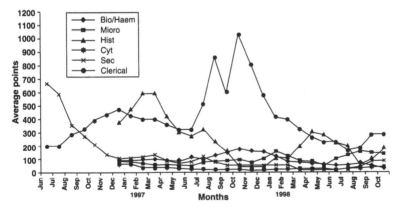

Figure 3.2 Monitoring sickness absence in a pathology service. Sickness absence was monitored in all departments using a scoring system which had been developed for the Rover Group. The score for each individual is calculated by the formula $S^2 \times D$ where S is the number of spells absent in the last 52 weeks and D is the number of days absent in the last 52 weeks. Following the introduction of this system, linked with appropriate management intervention, sickness absence rates were reduced over a two-year period.

What does a medical microbiologist do?

The work of a consultant microbiologist usually includes three major components, i.e. laboratory, clinical liaison and infection control.[8] Like other pathologists the generation of specimens links them to every ward in the hospital, but in addition infection control links them not only to the wards but also to every single area within the hospital. The microbiologist must maintain good working relationships in the trust with not only laboratory and medical staff but also nurses, pharmacists, Central Sterile Supplies Department (CSSD) managers, occupational health, catering managers, domestic services managers, laundry managers, the estates department, engineers and of course general managers. Outside the trust, daily contact will usually also be made with general practitioners, the consultant in communicable disease control (CCDC) and the local reference laboratory (usually a Public Health Laboratory). The wide remit of the microbiologist inevitably results in involvement in several different committees outwith pathology (Box 3.4).

Box 3.4: Committee work of the microbiologist

- Trust Infection Control Committee

- Drugs and Therapeutics Committee

- Health and Safety Committee

- Building/Planning Committees

Infection control

Each acute hospital should have an infection control team (ICT) which comprises the infection control doctor (usually the consultant microbiologist) and the infection control nurse.[9] The infection control doctor and nurse usually meet on a daily basis and liaise directly with management if a serious issue arises, e.g. closure of a ward. The rapid spread of epidemic methicillin-resistant *Staphylococcus aureus* (MRSA) has raised the profile of the ICT as it has affected most areas of most hospitals at some time. The ICT will be involved in the surveillance of hospital-acquired infection. However, production of specific infection rates is extremely time-consuming and may be available for selected areas only. A consultant microbiologist will usually chair the trust infection control committee and will in addition be a member of the district infection control committee which is usually chaired by the CCDC.

Clinical liaison

The microbiologist should visit the wards on a daily basis. This should include the intensive care unit, special care baby unit and any other high dependency ward. In addition the microbiologist should liaise with the clinical teams on the wards regarding patients with positive blood cultures (septicaemia) or other serious infections, e.g. meningitis. Close links should also be made with general practitioners to alert them to any serious infections in their patients, e.g. *Salmonella* or *E. coli* O157. General practitioners will also frequently contact the microbiologist to ask for advice for a range of problems, e.g. treatment and prevention of infections, advice for travellers and advice regarding return to work following infection.

Near patient testing (NPT)

Near patient testing is the term used to describe the testing of specimens outside the main laboratory. There is limited opportunity to carry out NPT in microbiology – dipstick testing of urine to screen for infection being the prime example. The microbiologist, however, is involved with respect to infection control issues and should ensure that there are appropriate facilities for specimen handling and disposal. Disposing of a urine or other fluids into a hand-wash basin is not acceptable practice! The different disciplines in pathology should be consulted with regard to training of non-laboratory staff, internal quality assurance, audit and the purchase of suitable equipment.[10] Fundamental decisions also need to be made with respect to the desirability of NPT versus rapid transport systems, e.g. air tube transport system and rapid reporting (computer links).

Audit

Each discipline is responsible for internal audit and external clinical multidisciplinary audits. For the microbiologist, audit may involve the diagnosis and management of infections in each speciality or infection control. An example of this corporate role of the microbiologist is shown on the case study shown in Box 3.5.

Box 3.5: Case study

Through daily review of positive wound swabs it became apparent that a number of patients of a locum surgeon had developed serious infections following clean surgery, although not with one particular organism. Audit revealed that these infections far exceeded those of the other consultants. Discussion with theatre staff revealed serious concerns about the locum's ability. This was brought to the attention of the clinical director of the speciality and the work the locum was allowed to perform was modified appropriately. The locum's contract was not renewed.

Audits should be used constructively as a tool to modify practice to improve quality. Audit of, for example, antimicrobial prescribing in conjunction with a pharmacist is useful in highlighting areas of inappropriate prescribing both for prophylaxis and treatment of infections.

Risk management and health and safety

There is a close relationship between health and safety, risk management and infection control. A member of the ICT should also be involved in the trust health and safety committee and the risk management group. Relevant information, e.g. the number of needle-stick injuries, should be brought to the attention of the infection control committee.

Research and development

The ability of an individual department to carry out research depends on the staffing resources and the interests of the individual, but as a minimum the assessment of equipment and reagents, and application of new techniques to microbiology should constantly be reviewed with respect to the possibility of local application. There must be constant development of better facilities for the detection and treatment of microbial diseases.

Education and training

Consultants should be responsible for ensuring that an active teaching programme is maintained within each discipline of pathology and formal teaching will extend to all the junior medical staff and in some cases medical students. In many district general hospitals the microbiologist is single-handed and trainees are not available. In larger centres, training of specialist registrars will need a structured education programme.[11] In addition, the microbiologist will be involved in the formal and informal education of other staff, including catering staff, domestics, nurses, CSSD staff and engineers.

Development of policies and procedures

The microbiologist will be involved in drawing up not only internal and external policies and procedures for the laboratory but also in policies which affect each department/ward in the hospital, i.e.:

• infection control policies

• antibiotic policy.

The infection control policies should be primarily drawn up by the ICT but will need agreement from the infection control committee to ensure that the policies can be effectively carried out. The link nurses on each ward should assist the local policing of the policies.

Each hospital should have its own antibiotic policy or at least an agreed antibiotic formulary to ensure that on a practical level the pharmacy department does not stock an endless number of antibiotics and that sensitivity testing can be performed to antibiotics that are available in pharmacy. The microbiologist can influence antibiotic prescribing by restrictive antibiotic sensitivity reporting, although this does not necessarily prevent inappropriate prescribing. The degree of control a microbiologist wishes to exert on the prescribing of antibiotics may vary, and pharmacy and the microbiologist must work together closely.

Clinical governance

As the microbiologist has access to each area of the hospital they are in a good position to be aware of poor quality of performance in all areas – clinical and non-clinical (see case study, Box 3.5). Auditing infection is the classical example for identifying problem areas, although this relies on the collection of accurate data which is extremely time-consuming. Infection rates alone, however, will not identify the poor performance of a surgeon with a high death rate (this may be evident to the histopathologist) or bleeding complications (haematologist), and the monitoring of infection rates in medical patients is more difficult.

What does a histopathologist do?

Histopathologists and cytopathologists are primarily concerned with the study and diagnosis of disease in intact cells and tissues. In most countries outside the UK the term 'cellular pathologist' is used to encompass the disciplines of histopathology and cytology. Traditionally, histopathologists have had a low profile within hospitals and most pursued a relatively solitary existence. Microscopy was carried out on tissue sections stained in a manner that would have been familiar to 19th-century pathologists, usually in surroundings that would have been equally familiar! Few histopathologists had much interest in cytology which was perceived as dull, repetitive work of limited value, largely (and often inappropriately) delegated to technical staff.

In the last few years both the narrow laboratory role and wider clinical role of the histopathologist have radically altered. These changes have been driven by a number of internal and external factors (Box 3.6).

Box 3.6: Recent reports which have impacted directly on histopathology/cytology services

- Establishment of cancer units and centres (Calman–Hine Report), 1995[12]

- Confidential Enquiry into Peri-operative Deaths (CEPOD), 1995[13]

continued

- Benchmarks for reporting criteria for evaluating cervical cytopathology, 1995[15]

- Review of cervical screening services at Kent and Canterbury Hospitals, 1997[16]

Establishment of cancer units and centres

This has required the development of multidisciplinary clinical teams with regular meetings that involve the presentation of histopathological data.[12] The histopathologist has become an important, and highly visible, member of the team. Histopathology reports are the single most reliable source of data for cancer registries. Increasingly detailed and sophisticated histopathological data are demanded.

Clinical audit

Participation in clinical audit is now expected of all hospital doctors. Histopathology is often perceived as the 'gold standard' test and many forms of clinical audit ultimately rely on a histopathological (or autopsy) diagnosis. Notably, the Confidential Enquiry into Peri-operative Deaths (CEPOD) exercise[13] was reliant upon detailed and accurate postmortem data provided by histopathologists. The autopsy is the ultimate audit of clinical performance and many studies have amply demonstrated that even the most advanced modern diagnostic techniques fall far short of perfection when postmortem findings are taken into account. In addition few clinicians will recognise deficiencies in their biopsy technique unless they receive information on the quality of the specimen obtained. Currently, feedback is given in breast and cervical screening, where formal clinico-pathological meetings are a requirement of the quality assurance programme. It is an important part of the wider corporate role of the histopathologist to ensure that appropriate and competent specimen taking occurs in all relevant areas of clinical activity and this should be adequately audited.

Research and development

The publication of the Culyer report[14] is focusing attention on the costing of histopathology services provided to clinical groups engaged in NHS research and development. All such activities must now be costed and nominal value attached to a histopathologist's professional time. Increasingly, research groups are requesting samples from fresh or archive tissue, placing additional demands on histopathologists but simultaneously enhancing his/her profile within the hospital as the 'gatekeeper' to valuable research material.

Education and training

Histopathology has traditionally been a consultant-based service within district general hospitals and few have regularly had junior staff. Trainees gained most of their experience in teaching hospitals where senior registrars have made a significant contribution to the routine service. The introduction of shorter, more intensive, training programmes[11] has meant that increasingly, teaching hospital histopathologists are finding their time taken up by formal teaching and routine service work, previously undertaken by experienced juniors. The teaching role of the cellular pathologist has also extended beyond the laboratory. Teaching programmes for specialist registrars in a wide variety of specialities now incorporate elements that require a contribution from pathologists.

Reporting and screening protocols

In the past, histopathology reports tended to be brief and, often, idiosyncratic. Increasing demands have been made from clinicians, commissioning authorities, cancer registries and screening quality assurance teams for detailed data presented in a uniform fashion. Minimum data sets are being developed for all common cancers and each requires the completion of a separate form by the reporting pathologist.

Quality standards have also been developed by the NHS breast and cervical screening programme[15] and regional quality assurance (QA) teams have been established to monitor these standards and ensure compliance. Histopathologists make a substantial contribution to both programmes and play an important and high profile role on the QA teams.

External quality assurance

External quality assurance (EQA) has come late to cellular pathology compared to the other disciplines in pathology. The output of a cellular pathology department is essentially a subjective clinical opinion rather than numerical data. Consequently, EQA in cellular pathology is not simply a matter of assessing laboratory performance but testing an individual histopathologist's competence to practice. The political sensitivities are obvious but tragic events in several UK laboratories and a general determination on the part of government to 'weed out' poor performers seems to have forced acceptance of universal participation in EQA by histopathologists.

Medico-legal

Many histopathologists spend a significant proportion of their time engaged in work for HM Coroner and a minority take a specific interest in forensic medicine. Consequently, more than most hospital clinicians, the histopathologist is familiar with medico-legal processes and may be a valuable source of advice for clinical directors and medical directors. With the introduction of clinical governance,[4] medico-legal issues are likely to acquire increased prominence. The histopathologist also has a specific ethical role in the use of autopsy-derived tissues. Traditionally, hospital autopsies have been a valuable source of teaching and research material for hospital clinicians. The use of such material is coming under scrutiny and the histopathologist in consultation with the hospital ethical committee may have to exercise considerable judgement over what may, or may not, be ethically permissible.

Risk management

As the events at Kent and Canterbury Hospital have demonstrated,[16] failures in cellular pathology may have a devastating effect on the hospital as a whole. In risk management terms, the cellular pathology department must now be seen as an area where it is crucial that the system is not dysfunctional. For many years histopathologists have protested that under-resourcing was compromising their work, whilst trusts, more concerned with immediate problems of waiting lists, overloaded casualty departments and unobtainable intensive care unit (ICU) beds have largely been deaf to such appeals. Post-Kent and Canterbury, all this has changed. There has been an explosion in the number of advertised consultant histopathologist posts, clearly reflecting the importance now attached to ensuring a safe and satisfactory staffing of histopathology laboratories.

Near patient testing/direct patient care

Histopathologists, wearing their cytopathological hats, are becoming increasingly involved in direct patient care. Fine needle aspiration (FNA) cytology, with immediate reporting, means that histopathologists are frequently seen at outpatient clinics, on the wards or in computerised tomography (CT) scanning rooms examining or taking samples. The role of the histopathologist as a 'hands-on' clinician is becoming recognised in many hospitals. This has undoubtedly increased the quality of specimens obtained and enhanced the profile of the service within the hospital.

What does a chemical pathologist do?

The chemical pathologist is involved in the study of the chemical and physiological mechanisms of the body in relation to disease. This provides the link between the practice of medicine and the basic sciences and employs analytical and interpretative skills to aid the clinicians in the prevention, diagnosis and treatment of diseases (case study, Box 3.7). This may be at the patient's bedside (near patient testing), within the acute hospital (on-site) or at a distance in collaboration with several trusts. Chemical pathologists also have a role in direct patient care in some specialist areas, e.g. lipid or diabetic clinics.

The chemical pathology service should be on the site of an acute hospital where the response time is crucial for effective patient management. At this level the similarities in the processing of the samples and advances in technologies of some disciplines (chemical pathology, haematology and serology) have made it possible to amalgamate the disciplines under a unified management structure. This has enabled more effective use of manpower, equipment and space, resulting in a more cost-effective service that is able to meet customer needs. The consultants will still remain responsible for their clinical areas for interpretation and advice. The consultative service provided by the pathologists is best located on the site of an acute hospital.

Box 3.7: Case study – chemical pathology facilitating a seamless service

The local primary care group, the trust and the health authority decided to consider coronary heart disease as one of the priorities for their health improvement programme (HImP). Chemical pathology played an important role in shaping the cross-organisational service plan. The following diagram illustrates the contribution made by chemical pathology at the different points of the HImP.

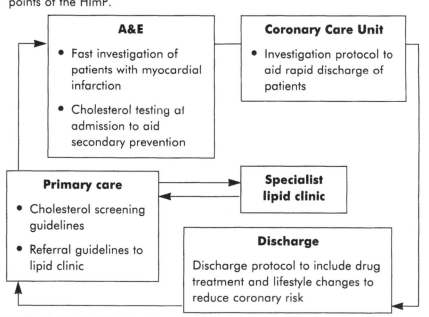

Remote testing of specimens is possible for specialist work. This service will benefit from economies of scale and scope. The type of testing that can be undertaken at a remote site will depend on the availability of an efficient transport facility and appropriate information technology. The offsite work of several trusts could be amalgamated to make this level of service more economical.

Near patient testing

Clinical management can be enhanced by NPT. Examples of NPT are blood gas estimation in special care baby units and ICUs and blood glucose testing in wards. There is also a place for NPT in primary care. The role of chemical pathology is to provide support in the choice of equipment and methodology, training and quality control.[10]

Clinical audit

This is a powerful tool in monitoring the total service in relation to patient needs, user expectation and clinical effectiveness. Chemical pathology has a corporate role in providing the appropriate service at the right time to help to reduce patient's length of stay and to avoid unnecessary emergency admissions. An example of this is the use of appropriate biochemical markers for the rapid diagnosis of myocardial infarction which prevents unnecessary emergency admissions and can help in the discharging of patients sooner from the high-cost coronary care units. Audit can be used to monitor the expected outcome.

Research and development

Chemical pathology plays a pivotal role in research – research not only in clinical medicine but also in the effective use of resources in the provision of an efficient patient-focused service. Here the discipline of action research is a useful tool. This is a process[17] where the approach to research is to combine theory building with research on practical problems. Action research is a type of applied social research where the researcher is involved in the process. Action research is a cyclical process which involves collecting data, analysing the problem, planning action, taking action and evaluating the outcome, and feeding back the evaluation into the start of the process.[18]

Education and training

The training of both medical and nursing staff is an important corporate role. This would include the development of evidence-based guidelines and the introduction of the principles of clinical effectiveness in the use of investigations.

Demand management

This is an important role of the chemical pathologist in containing the cost of health. This is achieved by education, agreeing on guidelines and intervening when laboratory resources are being used inappropriately.

What does a haematologist do?

Haematology includes the provision of a diagnostic laboratory service together with the clinical care of those patients whose primary disease is related to abnormalities of the blood and blood-forming organs. In addition, haematologists also have a clinical liaison role with other colleagues. In the UK, haematology has developed as an integrated investigative, diagnostic and clinical service. These developments have been reflected in the training of haematologists which lays equal emphasis on the clinical and diagnostic aspects of the subject under the guidance of the Royal College of Physicians and the Royal College of Pathologists. As a result haematologists have three primary responsibilities: clinical, laboratory and clinical liaison. They also may take on wider roles within an organisation.

Clinical

Haematologists have direct responsibility for their own patients. Within the speciality there is a wide spectrum of disease. Most haematologists will investigate and treat anaemias, coagulation disorders, inheritable blood disorders, bone marrow failure, leukaemia and lymphomas. Complex chemotherapy regimens are both chosen and administered by the haematologist. For the majority of patients these investigations will be performed and treatment given in the setting of either an outpatient clinic or a day-case haematology unit. The necessity for inpatient management has been reduced over recent years as a result of initiatives such as day-case transfusion and the improved management of infective episodes in neutropenic patients. There is still a requirement for inpatient admission, particularly for patients who require intensive chemotherapy or other procedures, such as bone marrow transplantation, or who require treatment for the complications of chemotherapy, such as infection during a period of neutropenia. For these clinical activities the haematologist will usually be a member of a medical directorate. In some of the larger hospitals, particularly teaching hospitals, subspecialisation in haematology is required, particularly for a regional service such as the management of haemophilia, bone marrow transplantation, haemoglobinopathies, etc.

Laboratory

The role of the haematologist in the laboratory will be influenced by the management structure which is in place within the pathology directorate. These issues are discussed in detail in Chapter 4. If the haematologist is head of department, he or she normally would be managerially responsible for all aspects of the service, including management of staff and the financial performance as well as the quality of the service. The haematologist has a role in the three stages of diagnostic tests (Box 3.2). The laboratory work includes a number of separate areas:

- Routine haematology – this consists predominantly of full blood counts, examination of blood films, ESR, etc.

- Blood transfusion – this is an area of a consultant haematologist's responsibility which is often underestimated. The consultant haematologist is accountable for the performance of the blood transfusion service within the hospital and for advice given to clinicians.

- Blood coagulation – involves investigating clotting problems of inpatients and outpatients and the establishment and supervision of anticoagulant monitoring services both within the hospital and increasingly within general practice.

- Special tests, e.g. vitamin B_{12}, folate.

Clinical liaison

Liaison with other clinicians, including general practitioners, regarding the interpretation of haematological results and advice on further investigations is another important part of the duties of the haematologist (see case study, Box 3.8). Within the hospital, a significant part of the consultant haematologist's duty is clinical

---

Box 3.8: Case study

A general practitioner telephoned to ask advice regarding one of his patients. This patient was known to have inflammatory bowel disease and had developed a peri-orbital cellulitis. A blood film report had indicated features of hyposplenism. The haematologist informed the general practitioner that patients who have hyposplenism are more at risk of infection with *Pneumococcus, Meningococcus* and *Haemophilus influenzae*. As a result it was indicated that amoxycillin would be an appropriate treatment. In addition, the patient should be counselled regarding risk of infections and should receive appropriate vaccination in accordance with national guidelines.

This case study illustrates the clinical liaison role of a haematologist in advising general practitioners on appropriate management of patients for conditions which may be picked up as incidental findings on routine blood films. In this case hyposplenism is a recognised feature of inflammatory bowel disease although it does not occur commonly. As a result of the blood film findings appropriate advice could be given to a general practitioner regarding management of both the immediate infection and the longer-term risks in relation to splenic hypofunction.

liaison with colleagues regarding their patients. This will include advice on the management of patients with clotting disorders on the ICU, advice for patients who are pregnant who develop haematological complications and routine advice regarding further investigation for patients either admitted as acute emergencies or as planned admissions.

Near patient testing

The haematologist should have responsibility for haematological tests performed outside the laboratory. The two main areas for NPT are the performance of full blood counts and tests required for monitoring anticoagulant therapy. For full blood counts the prime reason for near patient testing may be as part of a haematology or oncology clinic.

The provision of anticoagulant services as part of a NPT programme is an increasing trend. Traditionally haematologists will have organised NPT to support hospital anticoagulant clinics. With the recent development of small coagulometers, an increasing number of general practices are starting to monitor their own patients in-house. This development of NPT in general practice will expand following publication of the health circular in relation to the provision of secondary care within general practice[19] as health authorities will provide payment to general practitioners for the provision of these services.

Audit

Within the hospital the haematologist will contribute to audit performed in other specialities particularly if laboratory sources are being audited. The haematologist should, however, take the lead in audit particularly in relation to blood transfusion. Most hospitals will now have a blood transfusion committee which will be responsible for reviewing all blood transfusion policies and procedures and auditing compliance with them. The establishment of a hospital transfusion committee was one of the main recommendations from the recent Serious Hazard of Transfusion Annual Report.[20] As with the other subspecialities demand management should be a key role of the haematologist.

Development of a benchmarking system to compare clinicians' use of pathology may be a starting point in which inappropriate use of laboratory tests can be addressed.[21]

Risk management

Within haematology, two areas in particular should be addressed for risk management purposes. The first of these is transfusion. It is clearly an important area since if things do go wrong the consequences of transfusing the wrong blood to a patient can be disastrous. Therefore, under the auspices of the blood transfusion audit committee, risk reduction programmes should be in place to monitor non-compliance with protocols, etc.[22] The transfusion committee should review all policies and procedures in relation to blood transfusion at least on an annual basis. Another area of risk management is that of antenatal blood grouping and antibody screening. The haematologist can contribute to audit of compliance of established protocols with the obstetricians.

Research and development

Many haematologists have a strong track record of participation in multicentre clinical trials. These trials are usually concerned with the treatment of patients with leukaemia and lymphoma.

Education and training

The haematologist should play an active role in the education and training of all staff. This will include, for example, training of medical staff in the appropriate use of the laboratory. In addition the haematologist should be involved in the training of nursing staff in the management of patients with haematological disorders.

Development of policies and procedures

Within a hospital the haematologist should take a lead in developing a number of guidelines and procedures. First of all the haematologist should contribute to the production of a handbook for all medical staff using the laboratory. This will include guidance for use of tests and blood products. In addition, detailed policies will normally be prepared for anticoagulation. These will be based on national guidelines and should cover both prophylaxis and treatment of thromboembolism. Other policies in which the haematologist should take a lead are those concerned with the transfusion of blood and blood products as described above.

Conclusion

Like it or not, the pathologist has evolved from 'back-room boy' into a high profile clinician. External pressures and internal changes in the practice of pathology are operating to create a wider clinical and corporate role. It is important that the opportunities presented are grasped. The pathologist is a valuable resource for clinical and medical directors and their potential contribution greatly exceeds their traditional narrow laboratory role.

Key point summary

- Changes in the delivery of healthcare have increased the need for a high-quality, efficient pathology service.

- An effective pathology service is of critical importance to the overall effectiveness of healthcare.

- The pathologist provides strategic leadership in the planning and delivery of a clinical and cost-effective pathology service.

- Pathology services are available at the bedside (near patient testing), in the same hospital and off site.

- The clinical role of the pathologist and technological developments have expanded enormously in each discipline of pathology.

- The pathologist has a core operational role in a trust in monitoring and providing quality patient care (clinical governance).

References

1   Royal College of Pathologists (November 1989) *Codes of Practice for Pathology Departments.* Royal College of Pathologists, London.

2   Royal College of Pathologists (April 1992) *Medical & Scientific Staffing of the National Health Service Pathology Departments.* Royal College of Pathologists, London.

3   NHS Executive (1995) *Strategic Review of Pathology Services.* HMSO, London.

4   Secretary of State for Health (1998) *A First Class Service: quality in the new NHS.* Department of Health, London.

5   The Audit Commission (1993) *Critical Path: an analysis of the pathology services.* HMSO, London.

6   Shirley JA (1995) Are laboratories ready for market testing? *Clinician in Management.* **4**: 6–8.

7   Tickner T and Wallis I (1996) Path perfect. *Health Service Journal.* **106**: 32.

8   Mehtar S (1995) Review of a consultant microbiologist's work practice – an audit. *Journal of Clinical Pathol.* **48**: 1082–6.

9   Hospital Infection Working Group of the Department of Health and Public Health Laboratory Service (1995) *Hospital Infection Control. Guidance on the control of infection in hospitals.*

10 Burnett D and Freedman D (1994) Near-patient testing: the management issues. *Health Services Management.* March: 10–13.

11 Department of Health (1993) *Hospital Doctors: training for the future. The report of the Working Group on Specialist Medical Training.* Department of Health, London.

12 Calman K and Hine D (1995) *A Policy Framework for Commissioning Cancer Services.* Department of Health, London.

13 Campling EA, Devlin HV, Hoile RW and Lunn JN (1995) *The Report of the National Confidential Enquiry into Perioperative Deaths 1992/3.* CEPOD.

14 Culyer A (1994) *Supporting Research and Development in the NHS: the report to minister for health by a research and development task force.* HMSO, London.

15 Herbert A (1995) Achievable standards, benchmarks for reporting, criteria for evaluating cervical cytopathology. Report of a working party set up by the Royal College of Pathologists, the British Society for Clinical Cytology and the NHS Cervical Screening Programme. *Cytopathology* 6(Suppl. 2): 1–32.

16 *Review of Cervical Screening Services at Kent and Canterbury Hospitals NHS Trust.* (1997) South Thames NHS Executive, London.

17 Lewin K (1946) Action research and minority problems. *Journal of Social Issues.* **2**: 34–6.

18 Cunningham JB (1993) *Action Research and Organisational Development.* Praeger, Westport, Connecticut.

19 HSG (96) 31 (1996) *A National Framework for the Provision of Secondary Care within General Practice.* NHS Executive, London.

20 Serious Hazard of Transfusion (1998) *Annual Report 1996–1997.* Serious Hazard of Transfusion Scheme, Manchester.

21 Smellie WSA (1999) Evidence-based pathology principles into practice. Experience of a GP benchmarking study. *Association of Clinical Pathologists Year Book.* ACA, London.

22 HSC (1998/224) *Better Blood Transfusion.* NHS Executive, London.

4

Directorate staffing, management and organisation

MICHAEL GALLOWAY

Management structures within NHS pathology laboratories vary widely. Many are based on the clinical directorate model with a consultant or clinical scientist acting as a clinical director. Usually the clinical director will be managerially responsible for all the subspecialities within pathology. In some larger hospitals individual pathology specialities may have separate clinical directorates. Within the directorate each speciality will normally have a head of department who is clinically responsible for that service. A number of factors are influencing the traditional role consultants have in managing pathology services. This chapter will explore some of these issues and describes some of the management structures that have evolved in response to a variety of factors which are influencing pathology services.

Staffing

The staffing skill mix which is present in a NHS laboratory is shown in Box 4.1. Medical staff within the directorate will have been exclusively trained in their own speciality and will have obtained the appropriate postgraduate diploma (Membership of the Royal College of Pathologists). In some specialities, particularly chemical pathology (sometimes referred to as clinical biochemistry), clinical scientists will also have obtained this qualification. Clinical scientists have a role not only in providing expert scientific input into the diagnostic service but also will be able to provide advice to clinicians on the appropriateness of diagnostic tests and their interpretation. However, in view of their non-medical background the type of advice which can be offered will differ from that offered by a medical consultant. Clinical scientists currently are graded at three levels (A, B and C), Grade C normally being considered to be equivalent to that of a medical consultant.[1]

Box 4.1: Staffing mix in a NHS laboratory

- Clinical director

- Business manager

- Medical staff
  - Consultants
  - Trainees

- Clinical scientists

- Medical laboratory scientific officers (MLSOs)

- Trainee MLSOs

- Cervical cytology screeners

- Trainee cytology screeners

- Medical laboratory assistants (MLAs)

- Phlebotomists

- Mortuary technicians

- Secretarial and administration staff

The majority of the workforce in a pathology laboratory will consist of medical laboratory scientific officers (MLSOs). The grading structure for MLSOs consists of four levels (1, 2, 3 and 4) and was implemented in the late 1980s.[2] All MLSO staff working in the NHS must be state registered with the Council for Professions Supplementary to Medicine. A degree in biomedical sciences is now required for entry into this profession and for this reason the term MLSO is being replaced by biomedical scientist.[3] Most departments will have a MLSO 3 or MLSO 4 as a technical manager who will be operationally responsible for that department on a day-to-day basis. Medical laboratory assistants (MLAs) act as support to MLSOs. MLA training is usually entirely in-service and delivered by the MLSOs who act as supervisors. MLAs must always work under supervised conditions.

There are a number of other staffing groups within the pathology directorate who work in specialised areas, such as cervical cytology screeners and mortuary technicians. Pathology may also have control of the venepuncture service for the hospital and this will be provided by phlebotomy staff. There may be advantages, however, in devolving this service to users since experience in our hospital indicates that the users can develop a more flexible service which may include multiskilling in areas such as performing electrocardiograms (ECGs).

Management structures

Since 1970 there have been a number of circulars defining the management role of pathologists.[4-7] These circulars confirmed that the role of the consultant (or scientist of equivalent standing) was to be managerially responsible for the provision of laboratory services. In this role the consultant should act as head of department and be responsible for the proper functioning of the department, setting its priorities, and for the quality of the service provided.

In 1993 the strategic review of pathology services was announced and this was finally published in 1995.[8] This document, unlike the earlier circulars, challenged the role of a consultant as being in managerial charge of laboratory services. In this review a number of models for the possible provision of pathology services were outlined. As a result, the role of the consultant pathologist was, in terms of managing services, less clearly defined. It was stated that laboratory services should be professionally directed by a consultant pathologist or clinical scientist of equivalent standing. No recommendations were made regarding management structures, however, six areas were identified to ensure an appropriate consultant input into the service (see Box 4.2). Therefore the strategic review of pathology is one factor which may change the role of consultants in laboratory management.

Box 4.2: Role of the consultant in directing pathology services as defined in the Strategic Review of Pathology Services

Consultant input should be sufficient to:

- ensure that the process of producing the information contained in a pathology report is carried out to the required professional standard

- allow the consultant pathologist to determine the pattern of procedures that is carried out in response to a request for a report or opinion on a specimen

- enable the consultant pathologist to be in a position to monitor and influence demand for pathology services

- contribute to the strategic planning of the service

- enable effective multiprofessional (and multidisciplinary) audit

- guarantee appropriate and agreed teaching, training, and research and development programmes

---

Other factors influencing change include a number of technological advances in equipment, particularly in the areas of chemical pathology and haematology. Many of the analysers used in these departments are fully automated and are easier to use than their predecessors. Some of these analysers also allow for assays for a number of pathology specialities to be performed on one piece of equipment. As a result some laboratories have introduced multidisciplinary working with the amalgamation particularly of chemical pathology and haematology departments.

The private finance initiative has also had an effect on the way pathology services are managed. The private finance initiative did allow for a pathology service to be provided by the independent sector. Therefore in view of these factors which are affecting the way in which pathology services are managed, it is worth considering a number of directorate management models and how the role of the consultant in management may change.

Traditional model

The traditional model is shown in Box 4.3. In this model the clinical director of pathology is managerially responsible for all aspects of the service. The clinical director would be the nominated budget holder and would allocate budgets to each department. Each subspeciality within the pathology directorate would have a consultant or clinical scientist of equivalent standing who would head that department.

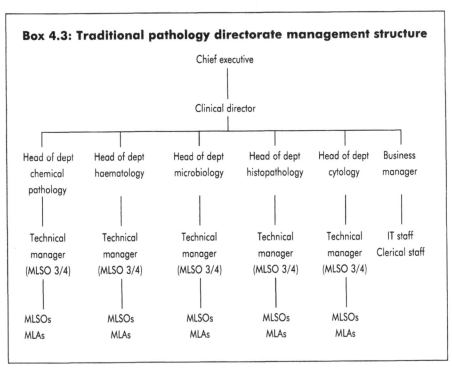

Box 4.3: Traditional pathology directorate management structure

Chief executive

Clinical director

Head of dept chemical pathology	Head of dept haematology	Head of dept microbiology	Head of dept histopathology	Head of dept cytology	Business manager
Technical manager (MLSO 3/4)	Technical manager (MLSO 3/4)	Technical manager (MLSO 3/4)	Technical manager (MLSO 3/4)	Technical manager (MLSO 3/4)	IT staff Clerical staff
MLSOs MLAs	MLSOs MLAs	MLSOs MLAs	MLSOs MLAs	MLSOs MLAs	

Role of the head of department

The head of department would be responsible for providing a clinical service and for the proper functioning of the department.[9] The head of department would be the departmental budget holder and would be managerially accountable to the clinical director for all aspects of the service, including financial performance and the quality of the service provided. MLSO staff in each department would be accountable to their own head of department for their performance.

Role of the business manager

Within the directorate the clinical director would be supported by a business manager. The business manager may have been professionally trained in pathology as an MLSO. Some business managers, however, may have a general management background with no previous experience of a pathology service. The post holder would usually be responsible for the general pathology services, such as specimen reception, registration, transport and management of clerical staff. In addition, the business manager would have responsibility for liaison with departments on operational management issues. It helps to avoid misunderstanding if it is clearly defined in advance as in which matters liaison occurs with the head of department or technical manager. These areas should be defined in a job description. Other areas for which the business manager would be responsible are shown in Box 4.4.[10]

The strengths of this model are that the role of consultant as head of department is clearly defined and the consultant can professionally direct and manage their own speciality. Potential weaknesses of this approach may be that both team working within each department and multidisciplinary working across departments would not be facilitated by this traditional structure. Some laboratories have an alternative structure where the business manager is managerially responsible for all MLSO staff and is then directly accountable to the clinical director. This approach may weaken the ability of the head of department to direct the service clinically. Team working within the department may not be facilitated. It is therefore essential that the head of department as medical manager retains direct responsibility for budgetary matters and managing staff within their speciality. It is important to ensure that there are clear lines of accountability and that the roles of the clinical director, business manager, head of departments and technical managers are clearly specified in job descriptions. This will avoid battles being fought over unclear areas of responsibility.

Box 4.4: Key elements that should be included in a pathology business manager's job description[10]

- Accountable to the clinical director of pathology

- Areas for liaison with head of department or technical manager should be clearly specified

- Establishment and maintenance of appropriate clinical, financial and personnel information systems

- External liaison with finance department, contracts department, estates department, etc.

- Responsibility for contracts, service level agreements

- Personnel issues, e.g. arranging advertisements, interviews

- Responsibility for general pathology staff, e.g. registration staff, reception staff

- Monitoring and review of performance of the post holder and scope of the job description

---

Multidisciplinary working and merger of departments

With the recent changes in laboratory technology a number of laboratories have introduced multidisciplinary working, usually achieved by the merger of departments, particularly chemical pathology and haematology. In our laboratory we have undertaken a similar process[11] and developed a management structure appropriate to our local circumstances (see Box 4.5). Within this structure the haematologist and the chemical pathologist retain management responsibility for their own standard operating procedures. A technical manager at MLSO 3 level has been retained for each speciality in order to maintain the professional input into the service. All other staff are now multidisciplinary trained and work on a partial shift basis to provide a continuous laboratory service. Within this structure one of the consultants acts as a lead clinician on a rotational basis and is supported by one of the technical managers also on a rotational basis. The function of the lead clinician is to co-ordinate activities of the combined department and to oversee managerially common areas in the department, such as specimen reception, registration, health and safety, and training. With time, no doubt, the number of common areas will increase and further evolution of this management structure will occur. We are currently reviewing how this model can be applied to the other specialities within our laboratory.

Box 4.5: Management structure following the introduction of multidisciplinary working and merger of a chemical pathology and haematology department

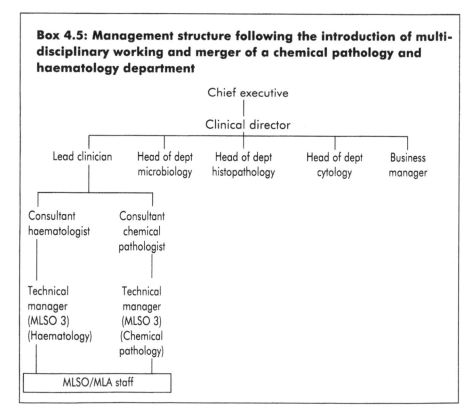

Some laboratories took the view that separate technical managers for each speciality were not required and the management structures were reorganised based around automated laboratory working, specialist areas such as blood transfusion and endocrinology.[12] We have taken the view that our technical managers are not trained in the opposite speciality and do not have professional experience to manage a combined area.

The strength of this approach is that in our experience it facilitates team working within the combined department. However, this type of arrangement does rely on good interpersonal relationships between all members of the team. If these were to break down the management structure as described in the box would be very difficult to maintain.

Clinical services directorate

Many hospitals that have introduced clinical directorates have had the problem of trying to rationalise the number of clinical directors for their hospital management team. Within the pathology and radiology services this has resulted in a combined clinical services directorate. This directorate will often include pharmacy. Examples of management structures that have been used in this situation are shown in Box 4.6. One option is for one of the consultants in the diagnostic services to act as clinical director and to be supported by a general manager. All staff in the laboratory and the radiology department are then accountable to the general manager. Therefore in this model the consultants are directly excluded from the management process. The role of the consultant in this circumstance would be to provide professional advice and guidance on his or her own speciality. This would appear to be a major weakness of this structure. For pathology it is essential that consultants can professionally direct their service and this model does not really facilitate this process. In addition, by combining the management structure across two separate areas devolved management is not really encouraged. It is also difficult to see how the principles of clinical governance can be applied within this management structure. The fundamental unit of management is the clinical management team. For pathology this must be each of the main subspecialities led by a head of department/lead clinician within the setting of a pathology clinical directorate. If the systems and practices of clinical governance are to be put in place it must surely be the responsibility of the clinical director of pathology who is responsible for the pathology service. For this reason it is difficult to see how this model can be effective.

If larger directorates are to be established an alternative model is to have separate clinical directors or lead clinicians for pathology and radiology and then to have one overall clinical director who sits on the hospital management board. The argument against this model would be that if the clinical directors are being paid a session then the costs of this model will be higher than the one described previously. Other models for a diagnostic services directorate are in use, however; if devolved management is to function, each speciality must have responsibility for their own services.

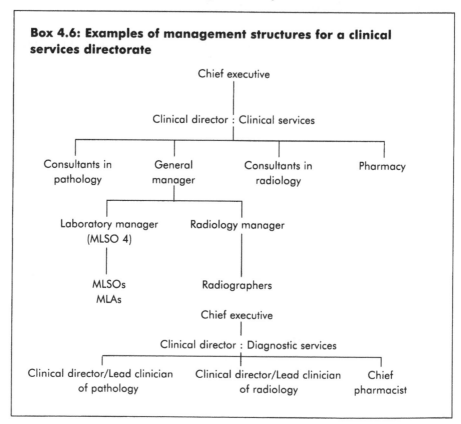

Box 4.6: Examples of management structures for a clinical services directorate

Chief executive

Clinical director : Clinical services

Consultants in pathology General manager Consultants in radiology Pharmacy

Laboratory manager (MLSO 4) Radiology manager

MLSOs MLAs Radiographers

Chief executive

Clinical director : Diagnostic services

Clinical director/Lead clinician of pathology Clinical director/Lead clinician of radiology Chief pharmacist

Private finance initiative

A number of laboratories have, for a variety of reasons, transferred the provision of their pathology services to the private sector. The first of these contracts to be agreed was between the North Hertfordshire NHS Trust and United Laboratories from 1 December 1994.[13] More recently a contract has been agreed between West Middlesex University Hospital and SmithKline Beecham Clinical Laboratories. The details of this transfer of pathology services to the private sector have recently been published.[14] The background to this transfer was that the trust board had decided to concentrate the hospital buildings on to a smaller site. Funds were not available to invest in new pathology buildings. After a detailed evaluation the contract for pathology services was awarded to SmithKline Beecham Clinical Laboratories. In both examples the consultants remained as employees of the trust while all other pathology staff became employees of the relevant company. In this model therefore the role of the consultant has to be redefined.

In the West Middlesex example a detailed agreement was reached regarding the definition of a consultant-led service, details of which are shown in Box 4.7. It is probably too early to say whether this model will be successful, since inspection of the trainee posts by the Royal College of Pathologists had not taken place at the time of publication of this report. In the report no mention was made of the success of this new organisation in recruiting two consultant posts which were vacant in 1997.

For the future this model would not appear to be a particularly likely option for trusts. The Royal College of Pathologists was successful in persuading the new government that pathology is part of clinical services and therefore would not be part of any future private finance initiative arrangements. However, it is clear that the present government is reviewing the private finance initiative and this matter is still under discussion with the college.

Box 4.7: A summary of the key areas of responsibility for consultants in the new SmithKline Beecham Clinical Laboratory[14]

Consultant responsibilities include:

- selection and appointment of staff

- prioritisation of work

- quality assurance procedures and policies

- test results

- introduction of new tests and methods

- equipment and reagent selection

- training, education and professional development of laboratory and medical staff

- accreditation

Medical advisory process

Each trust should have an established process for obtaining medical advice independent of medical management. The medical advisory process would normally be facilitated by a medical advisory committee (MAC) or a similar body. Within pathology one consultant other than the clinical director should be the nominated representative for the MAC. All consultants within pathology should meet on a regular basis as part of the medical advisory process. These meetings should be separate from the pathology management team meetings. The post of MAC representative, unlike that of a clinical director, would rotate on a regular basis between all consultants within the pathology directorate.

The directorate management team

The directorate management team would normally consist of the clinical director, business manager and heads of department.

Some directorates will have professional representation from MLSO staff on the management team. The team would have appropriate support from the finance department. It is useful to specify clearly the level of the support from the finance department, ideally in a service level agreement.

The clinical director should ensure that appropriate information systems are developed to support the work of the management team. These information systems should monitor key areas of performance within the directorate[15] and are summarised in Box 4.8. Once these systems have been developed the performance of the laboratory can then be benchmarked against other trusts as described in Chapters 6 and 10.

Box 4.8: Information systems which should be in place to support the directorate management team[15]

- Contract information (including service level agreements)

- Financial report for each contract

- Financial information
  - test costs
  - invoices issued and settled
  - expenditure by department with analysis of variance

- Quality information
  - test turnaround times
  - customer satisfaction surveys

- Workload data – this should be collected for each department and each contract

- Productivity data for each department

- Human resource data
  - sickness absence rates for each department
  - recruitment and retention information

Managing consultants

Clinical directors of pathology have an important role in managing the performance of all staff in the directorate, including other consultants. One area which the clinical director will be required to undertake is that of staff appraisal, which is one of the standards required for Clinical Pathology Accreditation (CPA).[16] There has been some confusion between the definition of appraisal, assessment and individual performance review. The Standing Committee on Postgraduate Medical and Dental Education (SCOPME) has clarified this area with the following definitions:[17]

- Appraisal describes a process which reviews and assists reflection on personal educational and job-related achievements. This process is normally confidential and covers areas including educational, personal and professional development together with career progress.

- Assessment is a process which measures achievement in college curriculum against set standards. This process is designed to inform the regulation process, i.e. the appropriate Royal College about career progress. Areas covered would include communication, clinical skills and competencies. Assessment is carried out both locally and by the appropriate college exam.

- Service performance review is a process which reviews performance as an employee against a job plan in the context of the local business plan. Within general management this process is usually referred to as individual performance review (IPR).[18]

The relationship between these three areas is shown in Figure 4.1. The SCOPME working paper also recommends that where there are serious concerns regarding the conduct or competence of an individual then these issues should be addressed outside any appraisal process. These proposals made by SCOPME are primarily aimed at postgraduate medical trainees. The usefulness of these definitions, however, can be applied to all staff whose performance is being assessed within a clinical directorate.

Therefore the role of a clinical director should include performance review for all staff, including consultants within the directorate. However, it is also clear that other aspects of an individual's performance should be reviewed as part of an appraisal. For example, appraisal may help an individual to develop the skills required within the role as head of department.

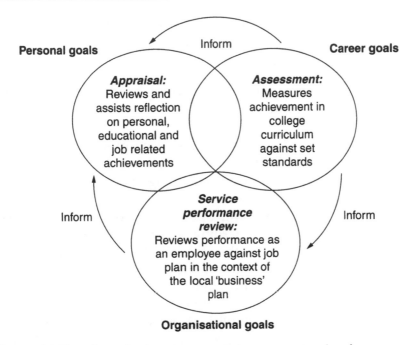

Figure 4.1 The relationship between appraisal, assessment and performance review in the context of personal, career and organisational goals (reproduced with permission from Ref. 17).

As part of the process of individual performance review the clinical director should ensure that all consultants participate in and achieve the required number of credits as part of the Royal College of Pathologists continuing medical education (CME) scheme. In addition the clinical director should ensure that appropriate continuing professional development (CPD) is available for consultants who wish to develop their role as head of department. There has also been confusion between the definition of CME and CPD. The recent SCOPME report on continuing professional development has clarified the situation.[19] CME is largely concerned with clinical, speciality-based issues whilst CPD goes wider than this and is a process that assists clinicians to:

- achieve personal and professional growth
- keep abreast of and manage clinical, organisational and social changes that affect professional roles in general

- widen and develop their own roles and responsibilities

- acquire and refine the skills needed for new roles and responsibilities or career development

- put individual development and learning needs into a team and multiprofessional context.

The Royal College of Pathologists has recognised that there is a large overlap between CME and CPD. As a result in April 1999 a revised policy was introduced which amalgamated both aspects of training into a new CPD scheme.

The Central Consultants and Specialists Committee has also published their guidance regarding appraisal for consultants.[20] The definition of appraisal in this document is the use of systemic methods regularly to review the work of senior hospital doctors. Two elements of appraisal are identified; first of all there is the clinical work of the doctor. Mechanisms for assessing clinical performance are not well established. In the document the BMA quotes CPA as a form of a peer review which assesses clinical performance. The second part of appraisal is the non-clinical aspects of a consultant's job. These areas would include job plans, service development, service management, teaching, training and research, together with CPD and the wider professional role consultants have in the NHS. This part of a consultant's workload should be appraised as part of a structured interview, possibly based on the annual job plan review. This review would be undertaken in most situations by the clinical director. Reviews of the non-clinical and non-managerial work of clinical directors would normally be carried out by the medical director.

Therefore this area of appraisal of consultants' performance requires some further guidance which will probably come from CPA. In the meantime what should directors of pathology do? In the first instance they should approach their local personnel departments. The personnel department will have details of existing appraisal schemes. In our laboratory we have used an appraisal based on management by objectives. In this system objective setting is the fundamental part of the appraisal, and performance is assessed on a regular basis against these objectives.

This form of appraisal is used to assess the performance of consultants and senior MLSO staff. A similar process has been developed at the Leicester Royal Infirmary (see Chapter 6). Another approach is assessing performance against competencies. For the other staff in our laboratory we have developed a competency-based system for assessing their performance. In this system we have documented the competencies which the staff require to perform their job effectively. Staff are asked to self-declare their performance against these competencies using a grading system. Then as part of the annual performance review, their performance is assessed against these criteria by the technical manager. Any gaps in performance form the basis of a personal development and training programme for the next 12 months. Using this format we therefore have a documented system of ensuring that all staff are fully trained to perform their roles. This is particularly important for those laboratories which introduce multidisciplinary working. A similar performance management system based on this approach has recently been described and it may be worth evaluating this approach to performance appraisal.[21] As mentioned above it is likely that some guidance will be issued by CPA and this will obviously influence the further development of appraisal for consultants.

Succession planning

The clinical director's contract should normally be for a period not exceeding three years. The post holder, however, should have the option for renewing the contract for a second term. Personal experience shows that it does take time to develop into the role of the clinical director and a three-year term of office may be too short a period to carry out fully changes that have been identified. However, it is also clear that two terms of office would be the maximum any one individual should be expected to perform. Succession planning is therefore important to ensure a smooth handover at the end of the contract. It would be reasonable to start discussion one year prior to the end of the current clinical director's contract. This allows time to identify other colleagues who are interested in the post and then if there are more than one, to determine what process will be undertaken so that one person is appointed.

Management training

Prior to taking up a post it is ideal if potential clinical directors identify areas of development that they require for their management role. This development can be undertaken either by networking with other medical managers in a similar position or by undertaking formal management training. Informal networking can be a useful aid to developing the management role. The British Association of Medical Managers (BAMM) Pathology Network Group is an ideal format for this. This group was established in 1994. Workshops for consultants in pathology have been held two or three times per year. These meetings have formed the basis for a useful network for clinical directors.

As far as formal management training is concerned, within pathology there probably are two options for this. BAMM has developed its own leadership programme which consists of three levels. The aim of the programme is to enable clinicians to gain a full and detailed understanding of management principles alongside developing and refining their interpersonal skills. This programme also gives credits towards the Sheffield Business School MBA. An alternative approach is to undertake management training specifically in relation to pathology. The Clinical Management Unit, Centre for Health Planning and Management at Keele University organises a diploma in management for the diagnostic services. This course is aimed at clinical directors of pathology and consists of three one-week modules linked with a dissertation. Each of the modules covers basic pathology management including operational management together with general issues related to the NHS, including health policy and management of human resources. Completion of this diploma allows for a number of credits which can then be transferred on to the Keele Health Executive MBA Programme.

Conclusion

Consultants in pathology have had a long tradition of managing both resources and staffing in their departments. There are now wide variations in management structures within pathology laboratories, many of which are locally determined and are very successful. With the development of new technology and other factors, management structures will continue to change and evolve. The development of team working across departments is a key factor in determining success of these new management structures. The role of the clinical director is essential in the management development of all staff, including other consultants. This particular aspect of medical management has been emphasised following the recent failure in a cervical screening programme at the Kent and Canterbury Hospital.[22] Although the report concluded there were failures in management at all levels of the NHS, of particular relevance was the lack of a clinical director for a period of two and a half years. As a result there was no clinical leadership within the pathology department concerned. In addition, the management roles of the heads of department and laboratory services manager had become ill-defined. This resulted in a breakdown in the procedures covering the quality assurance programmes. One of the recommendations was that there should be clear roles and responsibilities and reporting lines for all staff involved in running a pathology service. It is therefore essential that clinical directors are in a position where they can take full responsibility for the delivery of a high-quality and cost-effective pathology service.

Key point summary

- Traditional management structures in pathology are evolving as a result of the introduction of new technology and other factors influencing change.

- Management structures in pathology should facilitate both multidisciplinary working and team development.

- The fundamental unit of management is the clinical management team. For pathology this is the department led by a head of department/lead clinician within the setting of a pathology clinical directorate.

References

1 AL(SP) 1/90 (1990) *Remuneration of Biochemists, Physicists and other Scientists Employed by Health Authorities.* Department of Health, London.

2 AL(PTB) 7/88 (1988) *New Salary and Grade Structure and Revised Conditions for: medical laboratory scientific officers (committee A), pathology laboratory support grades, anatomical pathology technicians (formerly committee B).* Department of Health, London.

3 Institute of Biomedical Science (1997) *Professional Pathways for Biomedical Scientists: general guidance for professional education and training.* IBMS, London.

4 HM(70)50 (1970) *Hospital Laboratory Sciences.* DHSS, London.

5 HSC(IS)16 (1974) *Organisation of Scientific and Technical Services.* DHSS, London.

6 EL(89) p/171 (1989) *Management and Staffing of Pathology Services.* DHSS, London.

7 HN(90)18 (1990) *Scientific and Technical Services.* Department of Health, London.

8 NHS Executive (1995) *Strategic Review of Pathology Services.* HMSO, London.

9 Royal College of Pathologists (April 1992) *Medical & Scientific Staffing of National Health Service Pathology Departments.* Royal College of Pathologists, London.

10 Dyson R (1991) Business managers in pathology. *ACP News.* **9** (Summer): 4–6.

11 Smellie WSA, Galloway MJ, Woods R and Longmire W (1998) Introduction of multidisciplinary working in pathology – a successful merger of a biochemistry and haematology department. *Clinician in Management.* **7**: 216–20.

12 Harris RI (1994) The role of the consultant chemical pathologist. *Bulletin of the Royal College of Pathologists.* **88**: 19.

13 Anonymous (1994) Trust criticised for privatising pathology services. *BMJ.* **308:** 741.

14 Thorpe PA (1998) West Middlesex University Hospital pathology – laboratory service rebuilt by SmithKline Beecham Clinical Laboratories. *Bulletin of the Royal College of Pathologists.* **101:** 25–8.

15 Galloway M, Behrens J, Greig M and Shirley S (1996) *Management Information for Pathologists.* BAMM, Stockport.

16 Clinical Pathology Accreditation (UK) Ltd (1996) *Accreditation Handbook.* CPA, Sheffield.

17 The Standing Committee on Postgraduate Medical and Dental Education (1996) *Appraising Doctors and Dentists in Training.* SCOPME, London.

18 Institute of Health Services Management (1991) *Individual Performance Review in the NHS.* IHSM, London.

19 The Standing Committee on Postgraduate Medical and Dental Education (1998) *Continuing Professional Development for Doctors and Dentists.* SCOPME, London.

20 Central Consultants and Specialists Committee (1998) *Appraisal for Senior Hospital Doctors.* BMA, London.

21 George P and Cox RA (1998) Making it happen: successful introduction of a system of performance management into a pathology department. *Clinician in Management.* **7:** 142–7.

22 *Review of Cervical Screening Services at Kent and Canterbury Hospitals NHS Trust* (1997) South Thames NHS Executive, London.

Further reading

Austin N and Dopson S (1997) *The Clinical Directorate.* Radcliffe Medical Press, Oxford. A good introduction to management, including chapters on working in teams and managing people.

Burrows M, Dyson R, Jackson P and Saxton H (1994) *Management for Hospital Doctors.* Butterworth Heinemann, Oxford. A comprehensive textbook on management, including a historical perspective on the involvement of doctors in management and managing people.

5

Financial management

BARRIE WOODCOCK

Financial management has excited much controversy between doctors and managers. This friction is created by the transition of the medical role. Individual clinical freedom is being superseded by the clinical team resourced to provide a specified quantity and quality of service. Whilst this change has been caused by a complex array of social and technological factors, attention has frequently focused on financial restriction. Political control is increasingly being exerted through financial regulation and budget management has become an essential tool for those responsible for services. Controversy is being overtaken by mutual co-operation and dependence. The growing recognition that services must have an adequate quality specification has brought patient care back into focus. Financial management is now a means to an end and not an end in itself.

The objective of financial management in the public sector has been described as to provide value for money. Whilst this is clearly important, it is too narrow to be of use to a medical manager. Financial management is one mechanism through which the basic objectives of the directorate are achieved. Other motivational factors are important in determining the overall quality of the service but without the ability to purchase human and physical resource nothing can be achieved. The acquisition and distribution of financial resources is therefore a fundamental role for the clinical director.

Overview of financial management

The clinical director is primarily concerned with providing the pathology service within the agreed resources. The financial component of this management task is confined to the internal management arrangements of the trust and is termed management accounting. Some basic understanding of how this relates to the trust's statutory responsibilities is helpful in recognising the motivations of financial managers and in understanding the way accounts may be presented at senior management level.

Financial responsibilities of trusts

The public accountability of trusts is governed by statutory requirements and with respect to finance there are three statutory responsibilities for the trust directors:

- not to overspend
- not to exceed the borrowing limit (External Financing Limit)
- to earn a 6% rate of return on capital employed.

Trusts produce annual accounts and hold an annual public meeting where these are presented along with their achievements in healthcare. They are subject to periodic monitoring throughout the year by the regional office of the Management Executive. The frequency of this monitoring depends on their previous success in achieving the above targets. Failure to satisfy the regional office inspires significant fears and, at worst, may lead to job losses. The presentation of the trust accounts would include:

- a profit and loss account
- a balance sheet
- an income and expenditure statement

- a source and application of funds statement

- a statement of accounting practice.

Such accounts are for external consumption, and understanding of these is outside the scope of this chapter. However, some or all of these accounts may be presented at senior management meetings and issued to you as part of the annual report. (For further information see Cook, 1995a.)

Sources of income

Trusts derive income from the following sources:

- contracts with health authorities

- contracts with fundholding general practitioners (to be replaced by primary care groups)

- contracts with other trusts, private hospitals

- extracontractual referrals

- private patients and insurers

- sales of assets.

Expenditure is controlled through the allocation of this income to directorates and departments providing the services. This is relatively straight forward for service departments whose budgets consist mainly of their contract income. For diagnostic directorates such as pathology and radiology the formation of the budget is more complex and subject to substantial local variation. Such directorates will hold a variety of specific contracts but will derive the majority of their income from the contracts with the service directorates. Local variation arises in the methods for derivation of this income.

The pathology budget

The pathology budget may be viewed as a statement of the directorate's activities expressed in a financial language. It is an organic document in a state of evolution dating from the original introduction of functional budgeting to the NHS. As such it represents the accumulation of the results of negotiations and actions of many individuals, and probably contains fossil records of sequential management reorganisations. This line of continuous development arises from the discrete nature of pathology departments. They are geographically well-demarcated and their expenditure can be followed more simply than that of clinical service departments. Furthermore, activity renders itself quantifiable, although this may be misleading at times.

Successful management of the budget is but one facet of success in the management of the pathology service. In general, success means satisfying the expectations of others. In pathology this is particularly difficult. Key interest groups are represented in Box 5.1. Quality is a major concern for all, although perhaps less so for those principally responsible for finance. History suggests, and recent developments confirm, that quality cannot be sacrificed for financial expediency. This may be an increasingly difficult tension to resolve as the quality agenda becomes enacted in law.

Box 5.1: Interest groups in pathology budget management

Group	Interest
Clinicians	Quality
	Timeliness
	Cost for contracting
Patients/tax payers	Quality
	Value for money
Pathology consultants	Quality
	Professional aspirations
	Personal interests
Chief executive/board director	Quality
	Budget balances
	Probity/financial audit
Finance director/accountant	Budget balances
	Probity/financial audit

The structure of the budget

The pathology budget was originally a statement of expenditure against an agreed allocation of resources. More recently the resource allocation has been expressed in terms of income from contracts and other sources. The level of sophistication applied to the income section of the budget varies from trust to trust. There is a balance to be struck between detail of income and time spent managing it and this will be discussed later. It is simpler to begin with the expenditure side of the budget, which is consistent throughout the NHS.

The expenditure section of the budget

Each budget line represents expenditure that can be coded through the general ledger by a unique finance code. The financial ledger held in the finance department contains the full accounting records of the organisation. Through the financial coding all financial transactions are recorded in the general ledger. Staff expenditure is customarily around 65% of the total expenditure. Staff are grouped according to profession and grade. Their working time is expressed as whole time equivalent (WTE): budgeted hours divided by the standard contracted hours (e.g. 18.5 hours = 0.5 WTE for a standard 37-hour week).

Incremental pay scales present problems in allocation of resources. A common method is to allocate resources according to the midpoint of the pay scales. When staff turnover is low the proportion of staff who have reached the maximum increment rises and funding at the midpoint will disadvantage the department. Ideally the pay budget should be allocated on actual salaries and adjusted at the time of budget setting. Some budgets may include a staff vacancy factor which reflects an expectation that some posts will be vacant for short periods. This is reasonable but diminishes the opportunity to use staff vacancies to contribute to efficiency savings, which are required when the trust has a projected overspend.

Non-pay budget lines give allocations for consumables, additional staff-related costs and office costs. In addition costs of referred investigations, equipment depreciation and Clinical

Pathology Accreditation (CPA) inspections and subscriptions may be included. Much depends on the individual hospital methods of handling these items. The non-pay budget is decided on estimates of usage from previous years with increments for increases in workload. Its composition therefore reflects historical allocations and approaches taken for managing specific items, such as referred investigations.

Income section of the budget

The income section of the budget will vary in detail depending on how the trust manages its affairs. The major part of the directorate's funding will come from the contracts held by clinical service directorates. This may be allocated as a block resource or itemised in service level agreements with the service directorates. A block allocation may not be expressed in the income section and may be identified only as the difference between the income stated and the overall budget of the directorate. The other extreme will be a precise itemisation of the work done for the service directorates. The pathology directorate will hold contracts with fundholding general practices and other trusts such as community trusts. These will be superseded by contracts with the new primary care groups. There may also be allocations for outposted clinics, such as anticoagulant clinics and clinics within the hospital provided by another trust. Further NHS income derives from category 2 fees (such as family planning), mortuary fees (coroners) and those relating to section 58 of the private patients handbook.

Managing the budget

The role of the clinical director

Much of the management role concerns change. A complex array of evolving medical practice, changing management practice and financial challenge drive the need to alter our ways of doing things. Medical training and involvement in the medical community give the clinical director a unique perspective in prioritising such tasks and assessing their impact both on patient care and colleagues' satisfaction in the service. Hence much of a clinical director's job is in assessing and responding to the external environment and translating this into objectives for those managing the internal workings of the directorate. All of these activities have a financial perspective.

A team approach is necessary to manage the budget successfully and provide the service. Normally a senior manager, usually a trust board member, has responsibility for supporting directorates and provides a direct link to the general management team. An accountant from the finance department provides the technical skills for financial management. This is extremely helpful not only in costing proposed changes but also in suggesting ways in which resources can be handled or moved to accommodate the changes. The laboratory business manager has the vital role of implementing change and monitoring its progress. Establishing a co-operative and creative working pattern in this group is essential and will focus each individual's contribution on their strengths. This group should meet on a regular basis; a monthly meeting seems appropriate. There will be a dynamic interchange of ideas between this group and the directorate team responsible for delivering the service.

The budget cycle

This is an annual cycle and the three main stages are budget setting, budget monitoring and review. The latter is really a continuous process which culminates in a final review. The timing and methods may vary but these stages should be easily recognisable. There should be a calendar of agreed dates for this process which links to the wider cycles of strategic management, objective setting and business planning.

Budget setting

The most common approach to budget setting is called incremental budgeting. The previous year's budget forms the basis of the new budget. Two processes feed into this. Many trusts use a 'roll-over budget' approach. The previous year's budget is increased to accommodate pay awards and new pay increments and the non-pay section increased for inflation. For pathology departments there has been a consistent rise in annual workload and accounting for this is essential. Whilst ideally this would reflect the increase in workload for the forthcoming year, there is often a compromise and it may be that funding will be set at the previous year's workload. If the trust has a projected overspend, an efficiency saving will be set and the directorate may have to produce a plan of identified savings. This is the time to make adjustments between expenditure lines to approximate how the directorate is managed.

The second input to budget setting relates to planned developments through the business planning process. By this time the directorate should have agreed its priorities for the forthcoming year and taken part in the bidding process for funds. It also needs to have quantified the consequences of the clinical services directorate's plans. The funds agreed will then be incorporated into the forthcoming year budget. Whilst the process is conceptually tidy, there are often compromises made as the finance department reconciles the overall trust spending.

The advantages of incremental budgeting lie in its simplicity and efficient administration. The disadvantages lie in the difficulties in reconciling activity and funding, and consequently the link into the contracting process is rather crude. It may also hide changes in practice that have led to greater efficiencies. There is a tension between the needs for budgetary control from the finance department and the pressures imposed by changes in activity at the service level. What are the alternatives?

Activity-based budgeting directly links activity to finance both at the time of budget setting and throughout the year. The workload from each clinical service is quantified through a service level agreement or direct contracts, for example with fundholding general practitioners. The resources required to do the work are calculated and the financial implications derived. In practice, calculating predicted workload accurately is difficult, and agreements include incremental payments for work done above or below predicted. The attraction of being funded for work done is great but the process is time-consuming. Extremely detailed workload and costing data are necessary. Such information also requires careful monitoring. Two further concerns need to be considered. The first one is efficiency. Internal costing will tend to favour the pathology directorate or at least be seen to do so. Some form of external comparison or audit is important to ensure there is value for money from the service. Second, experience would suggest that overperforming services would not be able to fund the extra costs and an overspend would still be borne by the trust wherever this is allocated.

Zero-based budgeting requires that each year the budget is built from scratch. The objectives of the trust are first defined and then translated into activity. The resources required are then recalculated using historical data. This is a laborious process which is not normally used for overall directorate budget calculations. It is highly sensitive to workload change and efficiencies but requires considerable flexibility to implement. It may be applicable to certain areas, such as short-term contracts where renewal is unpredictable.

Budget reporting and monitoring

Regular review of expenditure against that budgeted should be undertaken for the following reasons:

• to assess achievement

• to identify trends

• to validate forecasts

• to identify key problem areas

• to review previous problem areas

• to identify future opportunities.

The objective is to provide the agreed service with the resources provided. The format and detail of reporting and the frequency of monitoring should therefore be decided on the basis of what is necessary to achieve this. Budget statements are often issued monthly and this provides a focus for monitoring meetings frequent enough to achieve the above intentions. The format given in Box 5.2 is standard as judged by example budgets from a variety of sources. There will of course be a list of all expenditure categories and a total. A negative variance indicates overspending and a positive one indicates underspending.

Box 5.2: Format of budget statements

Expenditure	Month			Year Date		
	Actual £(000)	Budget £(000)	Variance £(000)	Actual £(000)	Budget £(000)	Variance £(000)
Reagents	30	28	−2	85	78	−7

It is worth spending some time ensuring that the expenditure items are classified in a relevant and understandable manner and are therefore manageable. If this is not so, the exercise becomes increasingly time-consuming and thankless. Consistency in the financial coding of orders to agreed expenditure lines and the understanding of their composition will also facilitate efficient budget management. These roles are normally carried out by the laboratory manager and it should be possible to identify rapidly the cause of given variances.

Monitoring of expenditure statements is relatively meaningless unless activity levels are also monitored. Again the currency needs to be defined and understood. This task has become relatively easy in pathology departments since the introduction of computerised laboratory management systems. For the purpose of sequential monitoring the definitions of activity must be consistent and provided the categorisation is understood there should be little difficulty in providing information that is quickly and easily used. The difficulties that beset comparison of workload and performance between laboratories are not relevant to budget monitoring.

In practice, attention is primarily paid to variances. Staff payment variances should provide little problem. Budget setting is the time for active management of staff expenditure. On-call agreements, funding at actual salary levels and control of appointments to those funded minimise such variances. Unforeseen events, such as the necessity for locums, maternity leave and delays in appointments, have unpredictable effects. Non-pay variances tend to occur in reagents and consumables when workload is higher than budgeted and should be reconciled with the actual activity and its costs. Appropriate action can then be taken to seek further funding, reduce workload or accept the variance.

At the end of the year there will be a final statement. The regular involvement of the senior manager and accountant in budget management should mean this is an outcome expected by the finance department and the general management team. It is worth reflecting on what you want to achieve at this time. A great deal of effort and acrimony can be spent on trying to break even. What matters is that the directorate provides a service of sufficient quality and value for money. If this is achieved most interested parties will be reasonably satisfied, although the tradition for pathology overspending may be maintained.

Linking activity to expenditure

The link between activity and expenditure is fundamentally one of cost. Costing information should be obtained in sufficient detail to support contracting, evaluation of new methods, analysis of variances and the assessment of increases in efficiency. Costing is an art in itself and there is an abundance of methods. Again what is important is that the components of the costs are completely understood and the methods for allocation of fixed costs incorporate a coherent system of values within the directorate. We have found it particularly rewarding to derive our own costs and for them to reflect true costs accurately. By going through this process the composition is truly understood and the effects of change can be rapidly calculated. Many use commercial software packages equally successfully. Whatever the method, it is important that it is accepted within the directorate.

Specific issues in financial management

Defining activity within the directorate

The range of activity incorporated by the directorate must be defined so that costs can be appropriately proportioned. For example, the funding of direct patient care might be more appropriately managed through the medical directorate. If this approach is taken then appropriate proportions of medical staff and secretarial staff salaries should be transferred. This allows accurate costing of clinical care as well as pathological investigations. The purchase of blood products and their use is not within the control of the directorate (although prescribing may be influenced). A useful approach is to devolve the budget to the clinical service directorates and the management of it to the finance department. This avoids being asked to find the money for the blood product overspend from other areas.

Managing referred investigations

The pathology department acts as a staging post for some investigations. The costs incurred are again not manageable and increased activity will lead to significant overspend. It might be considered beneficial to devolve these directorates. The overall resources for these should, however, be kept within the directorate budget for the following reasons. Unlike the blood transfusion budget, there are usually several providers and service change may be necessary for quality or financial reasons. Furthermore, it stimulates review of the test volume and provides the resources necessary to develop the test locally should this become feasible.

Contracting with a defined group of users

External contracts with fundholding practices, health authorities and private organisations require an agreement on activity and price. Where historic data are available the activity can be estimated with reasonable accuracy and the price built from the cost. It has become standard practice to include a margin of error for the activity estimate (e.g. +/− 5%) within which agreed price applies. Outside this range a marginal cost becomes operative. This derives from the costing information and covers full payment for materials necessary for the performance of the test. Fixed costs, capital depreciation and staff costs are unaffected at this level of tolerance (e.g. +/− 10% outside agreed bands). In defining the outer levels of these limits it is recognised that fixed costs may change, for example more staff may need to be employed. A full cost or intermediate cost can be set. These contracts have been of value as the costs of excessive workload have usually been met and helped balance the budget. Smaller contracts where the workload is difficult to predict are better handled on a cost per test basis.

Similar processes may be applied to the clinical service within the hospital as cross-directorate charging or as service level agreements (see Chapter 8). This is a considerable management burden and raises the level of complexity of financial management. Whilst it may appear to solve the traditional problem of funding a rising workload, in truth the purchasers (health authorities) have cash limits and it may not be possible to fund excess workload (for example, emergency work which cannot be regulated). Many feel the increased complexity and consequent administrative time is not justified. Estimates of overperformance can be more easily obtained and costed from baseline data.

Introducing new tests or changing methods

Whether a new test is a new development or the replacement of previously referred tests, the approach is similar. Accurate, complete costing makes the process relatively simple. The presence of capital costs (depreciation and interest) in the non-staff expenditure lines of the budget enhance the flexibility of the department. The relative contributions of capital costs, staff costs and consumables vary with methods. Choices can be made between investment in new staff or equipment, between in-house testing and referral, and between methods of leasing or purchasing of equipment. A new test may require new funds and full costs should be sought through the business planning process. The costing of the approach is usually modelled within the directorate and if further resources are not required it can be implemented. It is always advisable for the directorate accountant to work through the costing independently prior to any decisions. This is always both reassuring and helpful and may give rise to promising new suggestions.

Key point summary

- Financial management is an essential support element for the directorate to meet its objectives. It is not an end in itself.

- Good working relationships between a linked senior manager, linked accountant, laboratory manager and clinical director facilitate financial management allowing the clinical director to focus on service provision and quality.

- The fundamental need is to balance the expectations of a wide group of interested parties and keep them reasonably content.

- Service quality is of prime importance.

Further reading

I have found the following to be very helpful. They have all contributed to the structure and content of this article.

Audit Commission (1993) *Critical Path: an analysis of pathology services*. HMSO, London. This contains extensive information and examples on costing.

Cook A (1995a) Financial accounting in the NHS. In: J Simpson and R Smith (eds) *Management for Doctors*, pp. 71–83. BMJ Publishing Group, London. An overview of financial accounting in trusts. Background information.

Cook A (1995b) Management accounting. In: J Simpson and R Smith (eds), pp. 84–100. *Management for Doctors*. BMJ Publishing Group, London. Budget management, including the history of budget development in the NHS.

Health Service Manager (1995) Croner Publications, Kingston-upon-Thames. Continuously updated. A practical guide and handbook for all areas of management.

NHSME (1992) *Finance for Health Service Managers*. HMSO, London. A self learning course.

6

Quality assurance

IAN LAUDER

As a clinical director you will have ultimate responsibility for the quality of service which your directorate of pathology delivers. You should be concerned because over the past ten years a number of high profile problems have arisen at some hospitals where an inability to deliver high-quality service led to serious harm to patients.[1-3] It is difficult to be certain as to why there have been quite so many instances where cytology and histopathology laboratories in particular have run into problems. The internal market as applied to health services was no doubt a major contributory factor. Staffing levels, equipment and resources were not increased at a level which matched expansion in workload. In the 1998 clinical benchmarking report for histopathology and cytology[4] more than 90% of laboratories fell outside of Royal College of Pathologists guidelines[5] for workload in relation to safe working practice. During ten years of the internal market there was rapid expansion of many clinical services, such as elective surgery and gastroenterology, which were perceived as good options from within the offices of an NHS trust hospital's contracting and marketing offices. Only rarely was any consideration given to impact on supporting clinical services such as pathology and radiology.

With the publication of the current governments document *A First Class Service: quality in the new NHS*,[6] the internal market has been laid to rest and the emphasis for the foreseeable future will be on quality. Traditionally there have been two main definitions of quality, namely: fitness for use and conformance to requirements. The users and their requirements will be varied. First of all you should consider the patients' needs. Their main requirements of the laboratory testing process will be:

- accuracy – getting the right answer to a laboratory test
- consistency – reproducible results wherever and whenever a test is performed
- timeliness – nobody wants to wait forever
- value for money – why pay more in taxes?

In general clinical users of our services will have a similar agenda and we would all like to hope that hospital managers' requirements extend beyond value for money. The challenge for you as a clinical director is to ensure that a quality service really is being delivered. In meeting this challenge there will be three main components:

- monitoring laboratory performance
- maintaining a good and modern infrastructure in your laboratories
- creating a quality assurance ethos within your directorate.

These three areas will now be explained in greater detail.

Monitoring laboratory performance

This is a complex process involving a wide variety of activities. These are summarised in Box 6.1.

Internal quality control

The real-time monitoring of analytical work by the use of internal standards and regular checks on a proportion of test output are a vital and integral part of daily work of all NHS laboratories. What perhaps is not appreciated by some clinical directors are the very significant direct and indirect costs associated with good internal quality control. The relative cost will obviously be related to the volume of work undertaken. These costs are a significant component of the economies of scale which the larger laboratories can obtain, particularly when a high level of automation is used.

Box 6.1: Monitoring laboratory performance

- Internal quality control

- External quality assessment
  - role of UK National External Quality Assessment Schemes (NEQAS)
  - histopathology and cytopathology

- Clinical benchmarking
  - Clinical Benchmarking Company
  - comparison of performance in a particular activity with other centres / organisations
  - College of American Pathologists – Q-Probes and Q-Tracks

- Clinical audit
  - often involves clinical users of the service
  - should be aimed at continuous quality improvement

- Individual performance appraisal
  - widely practised for technical staff
  - increasingly will be seen as a requirement for consultant staff
  - revalidation likely to become compulsory for all medical staff

---

External quality assessment

The UK can rightly be proud of its pioneering role in the establishment of good external quality assessment (EQA) in all UK health service laboratories. This was begun in the mid-1960s by Dr Mitch Lewis in haematology and Professor Tom Whitehead in chemical pathology. They realised that whilst good internal quality control could ensure good reproducibility of results within a particular laboratory, over a period of time there was a tendency for all laboratory results to drift away from each other – the phenomenon of so-called 'calibration drift'. The solution was to set up national schemes for all of the common analytes, involving circulation of samples simultaneously to all laboratories which were then asked to analyse the samples and return the results to the scheme organiser. The performance of every laboratory is assessed against the group as a whole and poorly performing laboratories are offered help to bring their results into line. By the 1980s all of the laboratory disciplines had developed external quality assessment schemes with the analytical schemes administered by UK NEQAS, and histopathology and cytopathology having been encouraged by the Department of Health's Advisory Committee (ACALS) to develop schemes for diagnostic histopathology and cytopathology.

The main impact on the quality of NHS laboratory work has been a considerable reduction in the variability of results obtained by NHS laboratories. This is perhaps best illustrated by reference to published results for haemoglobin for the period 1963–79 shown in Figure 6.1. The overall reduction in variability is striking and similar results could be shown for many other analytes. The total cost to a pathology directorate of participation in all current schemes is approximately £10 000 and, as ever, the clinical director may be called upon to justify this expenditure. The key lies in considering those laboratories which consistently fall at either end of the distribution curve. An apparently low haemoglobin could result in a variety of outcomes – more tests, unnecessary outpatient referrals, delays in elective surgery or discharge after operation. All of these have a cost associated with them which exceeds the cost of the original test and all of the associated quality assurance procedures.

The application of external assessment to histopathology and cytopathology has proven to be very controversial. Apart from the difficulties in how individual (usually regional) schemes are organised, there remains considerable dispute as to how substandard performance should be defined and what remedial action would be appropriate for individuals whose performance was suspect. With the coming of clinical governance and revalidation for all consultants, it now seems that at long last these issues will finally be resolved. CPA (UK) Ltd now has responsibility for the accreditation of all EQA schemes, including histopathology and cytopathology, and we can now look forward to a more uniform and positive attitude to EQA in these disciplines. Whereas with the analytical disciplines professional accountability will be monitored through the Joint Working Group on Quality Assurance, for histopathology and cytopathology professional accountability will

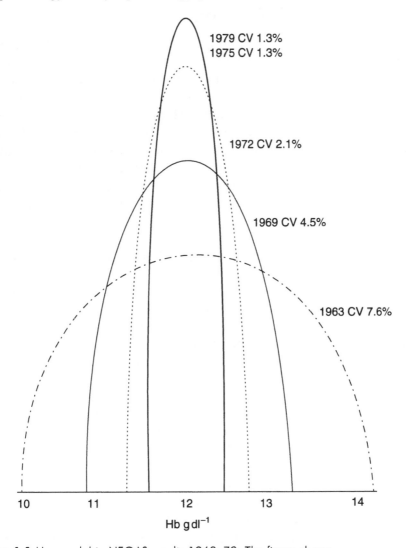

Figure 6.1 Haemoglobin NEQAS results 1963–79. The figure shows diagrammatically the change in the normal distribution of haemoglobin NEQAS results and the associated coefficients of variation (CV) for the period 1963–79. The data were kindly supplied by Dr Mitch Lewis to whom the author is indebted. Note how dramatically the spread of results was reduced over the 16 years' participation in the NEQAS scheme.

be through an advisory panel and the Royal College of Pathologists.

Clinical benchmarking

It has been a pleasure for me to visit numerous laboratories in the UK and abroad. Not one of these ever confessed to running a poor-quality laboratory! Some of these laboratories gave me serious cause for concern – excessive workload, cramped working conditions, excessive costs, suspect professional performance. In some instances the pathologists were aware of the difficulties but felt they lacked the necessary ammunition with which to attack the problem, whilst in many other instances the pathologists appeared blissfully unaware of the extent of the laboratory's poor performance compared with others. In both situations what the clinical director or head of service required was access to data which would have enabled them to compare their performance against current best practice in other laboratories – clinical bench-marking of their laboratory.

In general terms benchmarking seeks to compare performance for a particular activity with current best practice. For laboratories this would of course normally be with other laboratories in the UK but might well be extended to comparison with laboratories throughout the world. It is, however, worth pointing out that for some activities, particularly those concerned with management or process, it may be best to compare practice with other model systems in industry/commerce. For example, in dealing with tele-phone enquiries, how do our laboratories compare with organisations such as British Telecom or a railway station? There are many other examples that could be cited.

For NHS laboratories the most useful information is that coming from the Clinical Benchmarking Company. The pathology exercise is co-ordinated from Keele University by Professor Roger Dyson (discussed in detail in Chapter 10). It is now in its fourth year and for 1998/99 there are in excess of 100 participating laboratories. All five of the pathology disciplines take part, with expert advice being provided by an advisory group of pathologists and senior laboratory scientists. The benchmarking data are obtained from a detailed questionnaire which requests information on, for example, workload, staffing, test repertoire, quality and financial costs. After data processing a report is sent to each participating laboratory as a series of graphs, charts and tables together with some helpful comments. It is obviously important that clinical directors should be able to compare their performance with that of similar laboratories. To enable them to do this the data are now stratified as to hospital type and size. As with any investigation of this complexity there will always be some criticism of how the studies are undertaken and the interpretation of the findings. It is the author's opinion that good clinical directors really ought to be interested in the relative efficiency and performance of their laboratory. It is a pity that there are two-thirds of laboratories that do not take part in the studies, although it is gratifying to note that the number of participants has increased markedly this year (1998/99).

The College of American Pathologists (CAP) Q-Probes benchmarking scheme has now been running for over ten years. Like the UK Clinical Benchmarking scheme it is essentially a proforma-based data collection exercise. Q-Probes was developed by CAP to enable laboratories to monitor their performance and decide what changes might be necessary to improve that performance. The studies are more obviously clinically orientated and are designed to cover all aspects of the laboratory testing process from the original request to perform the test through the analytical and reporting phase to delivery of results back to the requesting clinician. In line with pathology practice in the USA the studies are divided into clinical pathology and anatomic pathology, and allowance is also made for hospital size.

In an individual study, laboratories are requested to collect data over a specified length of time. This information is submitted to CAP, who perform a detailed analysis and issue a report and a critique of the study as a whole, indicating recommendations as to how performance could be improved.

Until very recently there were very few UK participants in Q-Probes. In 1995 the Department of Health provided a project grant for a pilot study of Q-Probes in the UK. This enabled a total of 19 hospitals to participate in one or more of the Q-Probes studies. A final version of the pilot study report is still in preparation, but details of one study on urine culture contamination was published in the *Bulletin of the Royal College of Pathologists* along with a critique by Dr Mark Farrington.[7] Box 6.2 shows the results obtained by one of the UK participants and illustrates how the results are presented to the participants. Individual laboratory results are shown as a percentage and as a ranking percentile. Relative performance against other laboratories is shown in terms of percentiles and also graphically. Some studies are repeated (e.g. frozen section referral rates) so that appropriate changes can be put into effect and improved performance confirmed by assessment.

Box 6.2: Q-Probes 1996: Urine culture contamination individual report

Contamination rates	Your result (%)*	Your rank (%tile)	All institutions percentiles			Relative performance ++		
			10th	50th	90th	10th	50th	90th
All specimens	9.6	77	36.8	18.1	5.6	– – – – – – – ————◆————
Patient gender						
Male	8.0	58	22.0	9.5	2.3	– – – – – – – ——◆————————
Female	10.4	79	41.7	20.6	6.4	– – – – – – – ——————◆————
Site of collection						
Emergency depart.	–	–	33.3	15.7	4.5	– – – – – – – ————————————
Lab. or adjacent outpatient site	–	–	40.8	16.4	3.3	– – – – – – – ————————————
Non-adjacent outpatient site	9.6	78	42.3	19.3	5.5	– – – – – – – ——————————◆—
Patient age						
Less than 2 years	0.0	*	40.0	12.5	0.0	– – – – – – – ————————————
2–5 years	8.0	79	39.8	18.1	4.5	– – – – – – – ——————————◆—
Older than 50 years	12.6	66	36.4	18.0	6.2	– – – – – – – ———◆—————————

+ Higher percentile ranks indicate better relative performance (show as solid half of line).
Note: If you have less than 10 total specimens or your rate is greater than 70% for any subcategory, no rankings are printed for that subcategory.

As part of routine improvement of any system, CAP is now developing a new approach designated as Q-Tracks. As the name implies it is designed to provide a framework for a continuous programme of quality improvement. It was envisaged that Q-Tracks would eventually replace Q-Probes but it now seems likely that because of a large number of devotees of Q-Probes, the two schemes will run in parallel. Information about both schemes can be found in the CAP website (*www.cap.org* – see Appendix for contact details).

Clinical audit

It is now considered essential that all healthcare professionals should subject their clinical activities to regular audit. For pathologists the Royal College of Pathologists clinical audit department has prepared and published advice to all of its members.[8] The basic principles are simple: measure, evaluate, correct any deficiencies identified, and then remeasure and re-evaluate after a suitable length of time (the audit cycle). The Royal College of Pathologists maintains a database of completed audits and much of this information will be made available on the college's website (*www.rcpath.org*). Some audits will result in the production of new clinical guidelines, others will need to be performed on a regular basis to ensure their guidelines are being followed.

Much of the initial financial support for clinical audit has now been withdrawn at both local and national level. As a clinical director you will be expected to maintain and promote clinical audit from within your directorate's budget. Reference to the college audit database will at least avoid unnecessary duplication. One of the most effective forms of audit involves critical scrutiny of the work of pathologists by multidisciplinary clinical teams. This is now an absolute requirement for those centres seeking accreditation as either cancer centres or cancer units under the Calman–Hine[9] recommendations.

Regular audit will be aimed at continuous quality improvement through a series of audit cycles, at the end of which service enhancements will be made prior to the next audit of the activity (discussed further in Chapter 7).

Individual performance appraisal

Performance appraisal is widely practised for many professions but as yet has gained little favour with medical staff. This is all the more surprising since, within hospitals, individual performance review is almost universal for management and scientific staff. Since medical staff will be a very large component of the 'pay columns' on the pathology directorate accounts, it may seem curious that performance of this vital part of the pathology directorate is not always subject to regular assessment. Part of the reason is the tradition of 'clinical freedom' and the concept of 'premium inter pares' for all consultant staff.

The Leicester Royal Infirmary NHS Trust has pioneered an appraisal system for consultant staff as one of a series of innovations promulgated by the hospital's medical director. The scheme is known as the Annual Consultant Planning Programme (ACPP) and comprises an annual interview with the head of service or clinical director. At the interview the consultant is encouraged to define aims and objectives for the next year against a background of the consultants job plan, the business plan for the directorate and the strategic plan for the hospital. Performance is assessed against the aims and objectives defined in previous interviews. About 90% of consultant staff at the Leicester Royal Infirmary have now been through an ACPP and, in general, feedback has been favourable. At present the scheme has no real teeth, although it is easy to see how the outcome of such interviews could be used to determine a consultant's suitability for discretionary points or distinction awards.

The other potential major change to consultant practice is likely to come about by the endorsement by the General Medical Council of proposals for compulsory revalidation for all consultants. After the problems of paediatric cardiac surgery at Bristol, it now seems that some form of tightening up of professional self-regulation is inevitable and revalidation is a logical first step.

Maintaining a good and modern laboratory infrastructure

The delivery of a quality service requires adequate laboratory space with modern equipment and appropriate staffing levels. The best means of ensuring this is through laboratory accreditation and for NHS laboratories this will normally be Clinical Pathology Accreditation (CPA). Where serious deficiencies have been identified, most hospitals have striven to rectify these. It is not within the scope of this chapter to describe in detail the 43 standards which laboratories must fulfil.[10] It is sufficient to state that it is vital that all pathology clinical directors must ensure that their laboratories are fully accredited.

Increasing specialisation and automation will require new staff and new equipment. New technology and high levels of automated equipment are expensive. Clinical directors may need to consider that the maintenance of a high-quality, cost-effective service may only be achievable through reconfiguration of pathology services within a particular geographical area. A major government initiative can be anticipated shortly as currently there is a threefold difference between the most and least efficient laboratories in relation to total cost for an equivalent population. The internal market may now be dead, but there will be new pressures and new challenges that will have to be addressed. Service reconfiguration will be one of these.

Creating a quality assurance ethos

If you have already taken your laboratory down the road towards CPA, you will already have gone a long way towards achieving a quality ethos in your pathology directorate. What else is necessary? Movement towards harmonisation of quality standards throughout the European Community has led to a proposal for a new European Standard. This has been drafted by ISO Technical Committee 212, Working Group I, Reference No. ISO 15189. It now seems very likely that this will be linked to CPA. The main additional requirements will be the appointment of a quality manager and the production of a quality manual. For larger laboratories the quality manager will have a full-time responsibility, whilst for smaller laboratories it is envisaged that the role could be shared with other duties. One of the main areas of responsibility for the quality manager will be to ensure that all quality assurance procedures and guidelines are properly documented and kept up to date. This part of the job will be familiar to those laboratories that have successfully applied for ISI 9001 accreditation.

The advent by the National Institute for Clinical Excellence (NICE) and the related proposals for clinical governance[6] will accelerate movement towards evidence-based practice. We can expect an increasing number of clinical guidelines and more and more clinical benchmarking data. One interesting aspect of the proposals, which has not been widely debated as yet, is that medical directors will have access to clinical audit data. Because of the effort which has been put into the laboratory accreditation of all NHS laboratories, pathology clinical directors should be better placed than most to meet the challenges that lie ahead. The appointment of a quality manager as a senior member of the pathology management team will certainly help in ensuring that a 'quality ethos' is sustained in all of our laboratories.

Conclusion

Recent changes in the leadership and direction of the NHS have led to a welcome shift from quantity to quality. This chapter has summarised some of the more important aspects of how a clinical director for pathology can contribute towards the quality agenda. There is also the importance of professional performance of each member of the pathology staff. This is beyond the scope of this chapter as it implies individual rather than corporate responsibility. Clinical directors will need to encourage all staff, at whatever level, to maintain their professional skills and, with their hospital management, to provide the necessary support for continuing professional development of all staff. This is only one of several instances where all professional groups within pathology could, and probably will, be working together far more closely in the future. There are exciting challenges ahead for all those who take on managerial responsibility in pathology. Quality assurance will continue to be one of these.

Key point summary

- Ensuring a high-quality pathology service is the responsibility of the clinical director.

- All laboratories should be accredited by CPA (UK) Ltd.

- Clinical directors should monitor the cost-effectiveness and quality of their service by participating in the relevant clinical benchmarking studies.

- Clinical directors are responsible for ensuring that the appropriate infrastructure is in place to maintain the quality of their service.

References

1   The Scottish Office (1993) *Report of the Inquiry into Cervical Cytopathology at Inverclyde Royal Hospital, Greenock.* HMSO, Edinburgh.

2   *Enquiry into the Bone Tumour Service based at the Royal Orthopaedic Hospital Birmingham* (1995) South Birmingham Health Authority, Birmingham.

3   *Review of Cervical Screening Services at Kent and Canterbury Hospitals NHS Trust* (1997) South Thames NHS Executive, London.

4   Clinical Benchmarking Company (April 1998) *Pathology Feedback Report 1997. Histopathology/Cytopathology.* Clinical Benchmarking Company, London.

5   Royal College of Pathologists (1997) *Consultant Staffing and Workload of Histopathology Departments.* Royal College of Pathologists, London.

6   Secretary of State for Health (1998) *A First Class Service: quality in the new NHS.* Department of Health, London.

7   Lauder I (1997) Clinical benchmarking – Q-Probes. *Bulletin of the Royal College of Pathologists.* 14–17.

8   *Clinical Audit in Pathology* (1997) Royal College of Pathologists, Association of Clinical Biochemists and Institute of Biomedical Science.

9   Calman K and Hine D (1995) *A Policy Framework for Commissioning Cancer Services.* Department of Health, London.

10 Clinical Pathology Accreditation (UK) Ltd (1996) *Accreditation Handbook.* CPA, Sheffield.

7

Clinical audit

JUDITH BEHRENS

The pathology services of the UK have a deservedly high reputa-
tion for excellence. However, in pathology, as in surgery, there
have been recent high profile cases in lapses of quality which
make it particularly important for pathology directorates to have
effective mechanisms in place to demonstrate the quality of the
work that they do and to ensure its continual improvement.

This chapter defines clinical audit and outlines its evolution
within the NHS in the UK. Some suggestions for organising clinical audit within the directorate are made and an explanation given
of the recently published clinical audit assessment framework
which can be used to help improve the effectiveness of audit.

How clinical audit has evolved in the UK

It is useful to see how the lessons that have been learnt from the
audit activities of the last decade are influencing current and
future practice of clinical audit.

Formal clinical audit was introduced in an attempt to address
several important issues that had become a cause for concern
during the 1970s and 1980s. First was the growing realisation that
results of clinical research were not promptly translated into

everyday practice. For example, it took almost 15 years for thrombolysis to come into routine use despite good evidence by the mid-1970s that such practice reduced mortality. Second was the awareness that there was great variation in practice in the management of common conditions, from the vastly different rates of hospital referral by general practitioners, to widely different approaches to the management of common cancers. Third there was need to attempt to control the increasing costs of health. Different ways of managing patients led to differing costs; for example, different rates of day-case surgery.[1] The government saw the use of clinical audit by the professionals delivering care as a means of tackling these problems of varying costs and quality. It was acknowledged that many doctors measured and improved the quality of their care using audit techniques, and encouraging the dissemination of this good practice was thought desirable.

The 1989 White Paper *Working for Patients*[2] sought to build on what had already been achieved to create conditions which would encourage health professionals to make clinical audit voluntarily part of routine practice. Central funding was identified, and regional and district medical audit committees were set up to implement medical audit. In 1991 the initiative was extended to nursing and therapy professions, and in 1993 these were integrated into a single 'clinical audit initiative' involving all healthcare professionals in the health service. By 1994 the NHS Executive felt that the initial phase of stimulating the introduction of clinical audit was complete. The next phase was for local purchasers and providers to develop clinical audit further. Funds previously provided specifically from the centre to the regional health authorities were now included in regions' general revenue allocations in proportion to resident population and not ring-fenced as they had been previously.

The costs of audit activities were now to be met from contracts between purchasers and providers for undertaking a programme of clinical audits. It was intended that purchasers should have a more active role, for example it was recommended that 40% of clinical audit funds should be used for projects reflecting purchaser priorities. Purchasers were also responsible for monitoring the clinical audit programme to ensure that audit activities led to changes in clinical practice or the organisation and management of healthcare services, and thus to improvements in the quality of patient care. In turn from April 1996 the eight regional offices of the NHS Executive were required to monitor the performance of the purchasers to ensure that the objectives of clinical audit were being met. A large number of organisations and structures evolved to develop and underpin audit and related activities; by 1995 the National Quality Register identified 256 statutory, voluntary service and academic organisations.[3]

The direct costs of clinical audit initiatives were considerable, with the annual budget amounting to about £60m. In addition there were the opportunity costs which resulted from doctors and other professionals participating in audit. Time spent in audit meetings listening to an audit of someone else's speciality, with the awareness that the problems and pressures of everyday clinical practice were being left unattended, dulled enthusiasm, particularly if no visible benefit could be seen to accrue. A formal evaluation of the audit programme was needed to see if the investment was worthwhile and whether audit was achieving its objectives.

The success and failures of audit

By 1993 it had been shown that audit was integrated in clinical practice to the extent that up to 80% of doctors had had some experience of audit.[4] There was evidence that it had improved care in some cases[5] and had demonstrated its potential to improve care and use resources more effectively. However, many doctors and other healthcare professionals, managers and government felt that there was room for improvement. The views of the disillusioned doctors who did not find the audit process rewarding were not without justification. The formal evaluation of the audit initiative by the National Audit Office and the Public Accounts Committee[6] in 1996 found amongst other things that:

- many audits undertaken did not result in change in clinical practice. In fact in only one-third of audits was it apparent that practice had changed with clear benefit to patients, however, it was acknowledged that, in some cases, care had improved in a less direct and measurable way

- topic selection was not rigorous and did not address areas of importance

- there was a failure to implement findings.

It was little surprise then that the National Audit Office also found that not all doctors participated in audit.

The audit process from which so much had been expected was found wanting. On the other hand, the problems that it was meant to address had certainly not gone away. In the introduction to the 1997 strategy papers *The New NHS: modern, dependable*[7] and *A First Class Service*,[8] the new Labour Government lists amongst its main concerns, 'the slow introduction of evidence-based medicine', 'inequality of care across the nation' and 'failure to ensure the most cost-effective use of resources', just as had been the case ten years previously. Furthermore, during that time public expectations have increased, and there is greater awareness and intolerance of poor performance. Publicity surrounding events such as problems of the cervical cytology service in Kent and Canterbury hospitals[9] and paediatric cardiac surgery in Bristol[10] put the government under even greater pressure to act to prevent inequality and poor performance.

Audit had not delivered as much as had been hoped. However, the idea of audit as a tool to bring about improvement has not been abandoned. The Government intends to try to improve the effectiveness of audit, to enforce its use and ensure its findings are implemented. Many of the strategies of the White Paper have their roots in the recommendations of the National Audit Office report.[6]

What is going to happen next?

The Government believes that 'government and NHS have a responsibility to the taxpayer for provision of high-quality, cost-effective services'. It is their wish that 'quality will be at the heart' of the new NHS and that 'every part of the NHS and everyone who works in it should take responsibility for working to improve quality'.[7] 'The route to consistent, prompt, high-quality services is by setting standards, delivering standards, and monitoring standards'. They 'expect clinicians of all professions to work to a clear model of clinical improvement consisting of a continuous process of reviewing best practice, comparing it with actual practice and ensuring positive improvement is made'. In the White Paper this is called 'closing the improvement loop'. Legislation was expected in the spring of 1999 which will impose a statutory responsibility for the quality of services, and for the first time standards will be set for how services are delivered. Not only quality but also the assessment of performance is at the heart of the Government's agenda for the NHS. To assure the quality of their performance trusts will be required to have in place a system of clinical governance. Clinical audit is seen as one key component of an integrated strategy of clinical governance.

What is the relationship of clinical audit to clinical governance?

The purpose of clinical governance is 'to assure and improve clinical standards at local level throughout the NHS'. The concept is that clinical probity and quality improvement are monitored and reported in a similar way to financial probity and value for money. Trusts are required to put in place mechanisms to ensure risks are avoided and that adverse events are rapidly detected, openly investigated and their lessons learned.[7]

The practical structures for clinical governance will vary from trust to trust but clinical audit will generally be one of several groups reporting to a clinical governance committee which in turn will report to the trust board. The other groups will include those with responsibility for clinical risk reduction, complaints and adverse event investigation, continuous quality improvement and continuing professional development.

To oversee and support these new initiatives the Government has set up the National Institute for Clinical Excellence (NICE) which brings together many of the organisations previously involved in quality and audit activities. The board of NICE will be a small body of executives and non-executives with necessary expertise from clinical professions, patients, user groups, managers and research bodies. The council of NICE, whose role will be to review the board's activities, is made up of representatives of key stakeholder groups, such as carers, the Royal Colleges, academics, NHS service interests, pharmaceutical and other healthcare industries.

NICE will clarify which treatments work best and which do not, and the clinical guidance produced will be integrated into education and training, and also into audit. NICE will develop a range of audit methodologies that can be adapted for local use to support the guidance it produces. This will build on the work previously undertaken by the National Centre for Clinical Audit whose function will be incorporated into NICE. Importantly, it is recognised that to succeed in its goals NICE will need to build on and support new and innovative clinical practice at local level.

Monitoring the uptake of the guidance and audit tools will be the national performance assessment framework[11] and in addition there will be spot checks by the Commission for Health Improvement. National service frameworks will set national standards and define service models for a specific service or care group as happened for cancer services with the Calman–Hine recommendations.[12] Aiming to tackle about one topic per year it will also put in place programmes to support the implementation of its recommendations and will establish performance measures against which progress within an agreed timescale can be measured. There is a potential role for audit here to monitor adherence to standards of service delivery, although whether in the early years any service models specific to pathology disciplines will be produced is not known. Pathology will, however, be part of service standards for other discipline care groups such as the histopathological input required in the cancer services framework implementation.

How will pathology directorates be affected?

The General Medical Council explicitly states that as part of a doctor's duty to maintain their performance they must 'take part in regular and systematic medical and clinical audit recording data honestly. Where necessary you must respond to the results of audit to improve your practice for example by undertaking further training'.[13,14] The BMA's advice on the functions of clinical directorates confirms that it is the duty of the clinical director to supervise and oversee the clinical audit activities of their directorate.[15]

The structures and processes to facilitate audit activity are usually now embedded within trusts and their directorates. However, they must be reviewed and changed where necessary to ensure their greater effectiveness and their integration with other clinical governance activities. The clinical director must ensure that appropriate standards and guidelines are in place where possible, that they are being followed and that performance against these standards is being measured. Clinical audit has a vital role to play in assessing current patterns of practice and bringing about necessary changes and improvements. The clinical director can be expected to have a vital role in advising the trust board on which standards and guidelines should operate and where clinical audit should be focused.

Pathologists have for many years participated in a number of quality initiatives designed to measure and improve performance, and there is within the disciplines a well-developed culture of critical appraisal of clinical services and performance. These include NEQAS schemes, Clinical Pathology Accreditation (CPA) and other organisational audits. The point has been made that clinical audit differs from these because it looks at the whole pathway of care rather than isolated or single aspects, and requires continuous assessment and peer review.

How is audit defined?

The way definitions of audit have changed over the past ten years can be seen to reflect the changing values, ideas and emphasis which have evolved during that time. Earlier definitions were simple but clear.

The aim of audit is to improve clinical care by comparing actual practice with the general body of scientific knowledge and if necessary, by reducing any discrepancy between the two.[16]

The more complex definition of Working Paper 6 of the 1989 White Paper was educational and a useful working tool for professionals who had not by then a great deal of experience of the formal use of audit methodologies.

Medical audit is the systematic critical analysis of the quality of medical care including the procedures used for diagnosis and treatment and the resulting outcome and quality of life for the patient.[2]

The definition in the 1997 White Paper emphasises the need to consider the use of resources and to look at the effect of clinical activity on the patient.

Clinical audit involves systematically looking at the procedures used for diagnosis, care and treatment, examining how associated resources are used and investigating the effect care has on the outcome and quality of life for the patient.[8]

Types of audit

Clinical audit should be concerned primarily with outcome and the totality of the experience of the patient. However, the final outcome is built up of many components and these can be dissected and measured individually. Sometimes audits are thought of as those of structure, process and outcome but for pathologists it may be more appropriate to think of activities in terms of their access, process, output, outcome and use of resources (Box 7.1).

Benefits of audit

The patient should undoubtedly be at the centre of audit activity. However, audit has many other benefits all relevant to the successful management of a pathology directorate.

- Audit crucially can identify cost-effective practice and provide the clinical director, other managers and purchasers with information on quality.

Box 7.1: Components of audit in relation to pathology

Access – includes availability of test or expert opinion and information	*Is clinical advice available without delay when required?*
Process – includes patient ID, sample preparation, analytic performance, turnaround time and reporting systems	*Did the patients have to wait unnecessarily long for test results? Were results available in out-patient clinics on the day of appointment with physicians?*
Output – measures throughput	*Why has there been a 15% increase in requesting from medicine when activity has not increased?*
Outcome – considers the way in which laboratory results and pathologist's opinion impact on patient care	*How many women have developed carcinoma of the cervix having recently had a normal cervical cytology result?*
Use of resources – are there more cost-effective ways of doing things?	*Does the implementation of user guidelines result in reduced demand for tests?*

- As well as identifying and promoting good practice, leading to the development and implementation of clinical guidelines, clinical audit is educational.

- It can also improve team working and communication. Staff feel valued working as equals in the same project with consequent improvement in morale. The wide variety of perspectives and perceptions brought to the team can result in better decisions and be a rich learning experience for all involved.

Making it happen

Organising audit within pathology

The audit activities of the directorate should be co-ordinated via a pathology audit committee.

Setting up the audit committee

- An individual should be identified as responsible for managing the programme. This could be the clinical director or another member of the clinical staff with the necessary skills and training.

- Other staff and resources to support the leader should be identified, e.g. audit assistant, secretarial support and IT support.

- The committee should have a written strategy setting out its long-term aims and objectives and describing its activities and structures.

- Its relationship with the trust audit committee and pathology directorate should be identified.

- It should have a forward plan with short-term targets, timescales, deadlines, and assigned responsibilities and objectives.

- It should produce an annual report and evaluation.

Pathology departmental audit groups

Each department within pathology should have an active audit group involving representatives of all members of the department. Its members will perform departmental clinical audits but may also need to participate in regional audits which allow appropriate peer review to take place. This is particularly important where consultant numbers in a speciality are less than three. It would be expected that departmental and directorate audits would also take place in collaboration with colleagues within the trust, within the community and sometimes on a national basis. All these activities should be co-ordinated into an integrated programme through the pathology audit committee to which each departmental group should send a representative. In order to function effectively, appropriate resources should be available to these individual departmental groups.

Assessing the effectiveness of the programme

The clinical director can use the clinical audit assessment framework developed by Kieran Walshe and Peter Spurgeon of the Health Services Management Centre, University of Birmingham.[17] This may be of considerable help as a practical tool for diagnosing problems and identifying solutions for assessing and improving audit activities. The framework is further divided into sections dealing with assessment and those dealing with improvement. The full programme assessment framework can be used to review a number of recently completed audits, although some sections such as topic selection and impact may be more relevant than others. An overview of the programme assessment framework is shown in Box 7.2. The results can be used to guide the development of future audit.

Box 7.2: Programme assessment framework

Assessment sections	**Improvement sections**
Topic identification and selection	Management and direction
Impact	Planning
Costs	Support and resources
	Coverage and participation
	Training and skills development
	Monitoring and reporting
	Evaluation

Planning the programme

If the clinical director is not the chairman of the audit committee, he or she should have input into planning the audit programme. Time spent at this stage will be well repaid. The advantages of planning the prospective programme, say for a year ahead, are that audit activities can be:

- incorporated into the business plan

- co-ordinated across the pathology disciplines

- assessed against the criteria as outlined in the clinical audit assessment framework protocol

- assessed for workload and resources

- assessed for feasibility

- co-ordinated with other projects taking place outside pathology, either within the trust or with regional and national programmes where these are occurring.

Planning the project

It will be helpful to divide this activity into the following discrete steps:

- Decide on the focus and topic selection.
  - What general area or areas are going to be addressed and what specific aspect of that area to be tackled? It is essential when selecting a topic that the following criteria are taken into account. The topics should:
    (i) involve all stakeholders clinicians, clients/users, purchasers and managers
    (ii) address areas where there are obvious problems, or high cost, or high volume. Information systems should be used to identify potential quality problems
    (iii) be likely to lead to significant and achievable quality improvement.

- Identify criteria for measurement.
  - What are the standards which will be assessed? These may be national guidelines but locally produced standards are an acceptable alternative as a starting point if national guidelines do not exist. These local guidelines can be refined and expanded as re-audit demonstrates their effectiveness or otherwise.

- Identify methods of enquiry.
  - How will the data be obtained?

- Identify participants and population to be surveyed.
  - Who will provide the data? It is important to remember to involve trainees in the planning and conduct of audit as it is an essential part of their training. Other groups such as those in primary care should not be forgotten.

- Develop questionnaires, survey tools and audit forms.
  - These can often be provided by outside agencies / professional bodies.
- Draw up an action plan and identify and obtain resources.
  - Does staff time need to be identified or access to IT provided?

Once the data have been collected then it is necessary to:

- analyse and evaluate. Pathology or audit staff may perform this task

- draw conclusions. Generally this will involve the audit leads or relevant experts

- share results with those involved. Through minutes or presentations at audit meetings

- implement change through an action plan. What needs to be done to effect change? Who will be responsible for leading action for change? By what date should change take place?

  Note: In the past this is where audit has often failed.

- clarify and procure resources to effect the change if needed. It is a mistake to believe that most audits identify the need for increased resources. Often better care is less expensive care

- set a date for re-audit to see whether the changes have taken place and are producing the desired outcome.

These steps complete the audit cycle.

Although the concept of the audit cycle became familiar and it was a clear way of explaining the vital steps of clinical audit, it has recently become more common to refer to the audit spiral. This is a way of figuratively emphasising the need to go round the cycle repeatedly re-auditing to see if the changes implemented are still in place and producing the desired effect. If not, further change should be implemented and the process repeated.

Assessing the effectiveness of the project

In the same way that the audit programme can be evaluated for effectiveness, the audit group will find the project assessment framework useful in the ongoing monitoring of the projects.[17] A summary of the process is given in Box 7.3.

Box 7.3: Project assessment framework

Assessment sections	Improvement sections
Reasons	Objectives
Impact	Involvement
Costs	Use of evidence
	Project management
	Methods
	Evaluation

As has been emphasised previously, it is vital that projects are directed at identifying the outcomes of clinical care and the effect of care on patients. Ineffective audit misses the opportunity to improve care to patients.

What to do if results identify a problem

By its very nature audit will identify areas where performance falls short of the accepted standards. When this is so, action must be taken to make the changes necessary to improve performance. There may be many factors that contribute to poor performance. Investigations are likely to show that problems are due to process rather than to individuals. The clinical director has an important wider role as an advocate for all the staff in pathology in ensuring that working conditions, resources, education and training, staffing and workload ratios are such that all tasks can be performed to high standards. In some cases audit will identify the need for doctors or other members of staff to undergo further training and the clinical director must support and facilitate this.

If the problem is more serious then rarely, with the assistance of the trust clinical governance group, it may be necessary to prevent an individual from working whilst investigations are in place. The assistance of outside experts is essential in these circumstances and the advice of the Royal College of Pathologists should be sought. The trust clinical governance group and the college will advise on whether further outside agencies would need to be involved.

Ingredients of success

The clinical director will share the aims of the Government of delivering high-quality, cost-effective care but the Government themselves recognise that it will not be easy to achieve. They state that 'the drive to place quality at the heart of the NHS is not about ticking checklists but about changing attitudes'. They acknowledge it will require strong leadership at local level, and that local ownership is vital to the success of implementation.[8] The clinical director clearly has a key role of engaging and motivating the members of his or her directorate to take up the challenge of delivering quality improvement. Effective clinical audit is one important tool that can be used to achieve that goal.

Key point summary

- Clinical audit should be part of a pathology directorate routine activity.

- The clinical director should nominate an individual pathologist to lead and manage the pathology audit programme.

- The directorate should establish an audit committee.

- The effectiveness of audit programmes should be evaluated using published criteria.

- Clinical audit will form an integral part of clinical governance.

References

1   Hopkins A (1995) Some reservations about clinical guidelines. *Archives of Disease in Childhood.* **72**: 70–5.

2   Department of Health (1989) *Working for Patients*. HMSO, London.

3   EL [95] 74 (1995) *The Quality Register*. NHS Executive, London.

4   Mann D (1996) *Clinical Audit in the NHS. A Position Statement*. Health Care Directorate, London.

5   Department of Health (1993) *The Evolution of Clinical Audit*. NHS Management Executive, London.

6   Report by the Comptroller and Auditor General (1995) *Clinical Audit in England*. HC 27, Session 1995–96.

7   Secretary of State for Health (1997) *The New NHS: modern, dependable*. HMSO, London.

8   Secretary of State for Health (1998) *A First Class Service: quality in the new NHS*. Department of Health, London.

9   *Review of Cervical Screening Services at Kent and Canterbury Hospitals NHS Trust*. South Thames NHS Executive, London.

10 Horton R (1998) How should doctors respond to the GMC's judgement on Bristol. *Lancet*. **351**: 1900–1.

11 EL [98] 4 (1998) *A National Framework for Assessing Performance*. NHS Executive, London.

12 Calman K and Hine D (1995) *A Policy Framework for Commissioning Cancer Services*. Department of Health, London.

13 GMC (1998) *Good Medical Practice*. General Medical Council, London.

14 GMC (1998) *Maintaining Good Medical Practice*. General Medical Council, London.

15 Central Consultants and Specialists Committee (1990) *Guidance on Clinical Directorates*. BMA, London.

16 Shaw C (1989) *Medical Audit – A Hospital Handbook* (2e), 1.1. King's Fund Centre, London.

17 Walshe K and Spurgeon P (1998) *Clinical Audit Assessment Framework, HSMC Handbook*, Series 24. Health Services Management Centre, University of Birmingham.

Further reading

Report of the Standing Medical Advisory Committee (1990) *The Quality of Medical Care.* HMSO, London.

Clinical Audit in Pathology (1997) The Royal College of Pathologists, Association of Clinical Biochemists and Institute of Biomedical Science.

8

Service level agreements

MICHAEL GALLOWAY

Pathology laboratories will have a number of contracts with users. In the past these will have been primarily negotiated with fund-holding general practitioners or health authorities on behalf of non-fundholding general practitioners. In the future these contracts will be developed with primary care groups which may or may not be separate trusts. Generally these contracts will be arranged primarily through the contracts department in the trust. Less well developed are arrangements for internal contracts within a hospital. These internal contracts are referred to as service level agreements (SLAs). A service level agreement is an agreement between two departments in a hospital where one is providing a service to the other. Typically these agreements are between the bed-occupying clinical directorates and the pathology and radiology services.

The purpose of a pathology SLA is to allow the pathology service to focus on the requirements of its customers, i.e. users of the laboratory service. The SLA should also allow for a partnership to form between the pathology laboratory and users. The agreement should provide:

- the laboratory users with a guarantee of service provision and performance

- the users with a clearer understanding of the needs of the laboratory

- a mechanism to accommodate service development or change within the user's clinical directorate.

Need for service level agreements

When SLAs were introduced into our hospital in 1995, discussions with clinical directors and general managers showed that they had a lack of understanding of their requirements from the pathology service. In addition, observations at departmental clinical meetings indicated that the requirements of the pathology service were rapidly changing. Turnaround times for routine pathology tests needed to be significantly reduced. This was as a result of a number of developments, including an increasing emphasis on day-case surgery and one-stop diagnostic clinics, together with the opening of a medical admissions ward and the resultant shorter length of stay for medical emergencies.

This change in need from the pathology service had never been communicated by clinicians or general managers directly to any of the pathologists. As a result there was a risk that the pathology service would seem to be performing poorly and not meeting clinical expectations. In this situation SLAs do allow the pathology service to take a proactive role and to lead discussions related to these changes in service expectations.

Another reason for producing SLAs is to support the development of financial control at directorate level. Experience in the British Association of Medical Managers (BAMM) Pathology Network Group, however, does not support this as a prime reason for introducing SLAs.[1] In those hospitals in which SLAs had been introduced purely for financial reasons, budgetary control did not follow and SLAs as a result were discontinued. In addition, there are significant transaction costs in setting up a detailed invoicing system for each clinical directorate if full cross-charging for pathology services is to be introduced. If financial monitoring is part of a SLA there should be some debate as to whether the full budget costs for that activity are devolved or only part of that budget, e.g. variable costs. There are pros and cons for either approach. The disadvantage of devolving the total budget is that the user has no control over many parts of the laboratory budget, for example, overhead costs, staff costs, etc. This may result in the user becoming disillusioned by an inability to achieve financial savings if activity is reduced. In some areas variable costs are high, for example blood products. This may be an easier budget to devolve since activity is almost directly related to expenditure. Therefore it would seem appropriate to introduce cross-charging in areas where activity would be largely related to expenditure, for example blood products, referred out tests and other tests with high variable costs.

Process of introducing service level agreements

A pilot study in one area may be a useful way of introducing SLAs. The area to be chosen could be one in which there are known problems, for example regular complaints, or one in which a specific type of service is required, for example an intensive care unit. The laboratory should take the lead in the development of the process. A project group should be established with representation from the laboratory by the clinical director, laboratory business manager and other consultants as appropriate, together with users, for example clinical director, nurse manager, nursing staff and junior doctors. A draft SLA should be prepared by the laboratory. This draft should then form the basis for discussion with the users. Drawing on lessons from the pilot study SLAs can then be developed for other specialities.

Issues to be included in the service level agreement

The areas which should be included in the SLA are shown in Box 8.1. These can be divided into the following.

General issues

A number of general issues will need to be clearly defined. The length of the agreement with a review date, method for the charging of any tests or blood products and an estimation for inflation should all be specified in the agreement. The method for monitoring and liaising should also be specified as should any arbitration process if this is required. Other general areas which need to be detailed include transport of samples to the laboratory and transmission of results back to the user, whether this is by paper copy or electronic transmission.

Box 8.1: Items which should be included in a pathology service level agreement

General
      Objectives
      Duration
      Review and renewal period
      Method of arbitration

Service specification
      Range and volume of tests
      Provision and support of near patient testing
      Infection control
      Availability of clinical advice from consultants
      Contribution to teaching and training

Quality standards
      CPA (UK) Ltd
      Turnaround times – emergency
                    – urgent
                    – routine
      Development and monitoring of protocols

Laboratory requirements
      Adequate completion of patient identification
      Timing of collection and delivery of samples to the laboratory

Specification of services

A clear specification of the range and volume of tests to be provided for each speciality is required. The range of services will reflect the wider role which the clinical pathology service should provide. These would include advice on infection control, policies for near patient testing including purchasing and maintenance of equipment, staff training and quality control. The availability of clinical advice from consultants should be specified so that users are aware, particularly for out of hours, of the availability of consultants in pathology.

One of the main areas to be addressed in any SLA is the development of quality standards. First, the laboratory should be accredited by a recognised accreditation scheme. While there are a number of systems available, Clinical Pathology Accreditation (CPA) would appear to be the most appropriate for laboratories in the UK. One of the main areas of quality from the user's point of view is turnaround times for laboratory tests. There should be a clear understanding of the definition which is used to specify turnaround times. The turnaround times may include the total time from test ordering to the time the test result is received by the clinician. Monitoring of this turnaround time will be more difficult on a routine basis. A more realistic definition is to specify the time from receipt of the sample in the laboratory to the time that the result is available, either on paper or electronic form. Monitoring of this time is relatively straightforward from data produced by the laboratory computer. Other parts of the turnaround time can then be monitored by sampling audits which can be carried out on a regular basis.

A useful starting point when writing a SLA for pathology services, particularly in relation to turnaround times, is the specification for laboratory services produced by the Scottish Office[2] and KPMG Management Consulting.[3] Using this document as a template we prepared standards for turnaround times for each subspeciality within pathology. As an example, Box 8.2 shows a summary of our definition of turnaround times for haematology tests.

As part of the agreement, users will need to be educated regarding the ability of the laboratory to produce rapid turnaround

Box 8.2: A summary of the standards for turnaround times for haematology

Emergency: Results will be available within 30 minutes of arrival of specimens 98% of the time, and within 45 minutes 100% of the time. Blood transfusion cross-matching should take 30 minutes to carry out and results should be available in 45 minutes 98% of the time. Results will be notified to the user either by telephone or by the ward computer link on all occasions, as will any difficulties or delays. It is anticipated that the emergency service will generally only apply in the case of:

- full blood counts in clinical emergencies
- coagulation screens (PT, APT, fibrinogen, FDP) required in clinical emergencies
- blood transfusion services in clinical emergencies

For these specimens the laboratory will expect the sample to arrive within 15 minutes of collection of the sample

Priority: All inpatient samples for the investigations listed below will be categorised as priority. The turnaround time for these samples will be 1 hour in 98% of occasions, defined as the time from receipt of the sample to the time the result is available via the ward computer link and within 2 hours in 100% of occasions

This classification will generally apply to the following investigations:

- full blood counts
- anticoagulant control tests
- blood transfusion services in urgent clinical situations

Routine: Routine requests are divided between those requiring a one working day turnaround time and those which for technical or economic reasons can only be processed to a longer time scale. Results must be available within the stated time schedule 98% of the time

times. These will be affected by either the technology used, for example culture for bacterial growth or batch size since it may be uneconomic to run small batches. SLAs also offer the opportunity for the laboratory to agree some protocols for testing with users, for example blood group and antibody screening in antenatal patients, blood ordering schedules for planned surgical cases, etc.

Laboratory requirements

Within the SLA, agreement should be reached with users over the requirements and standards they should achieve when using the pathology services. For example, agreement should be reached regarding the minimum patient identification required when request forms are completed. Similarly an agreement should also be reached over the timing of collection and delivery of samples to the laboratory.

Monitoring of service level agreements

Monitoring of SLAs is a key aspect to ensure their successful implementation.

Monitoring turnaround times

Monitoring turnaround times gives the laboratory an opportunity to identify areas for improved performance. The data should be generated from routine reports produced by the laboratory computer. This will be feasible if the turnaround time is a measure from the time the sample was received to the time the report was generated. The monitoring system in use in our laboratory reports percentage of samples which have achieved the specified turn-around times. Within the monitoring system it is probably not necessary to monitor every test performed by the laboratory. It is important, however, to pick out a range of appropriate tests for each category of turnaround times. In the spreadsheet (Box 8.3) that we use for summarising the results we use a colour coding system. Results that are reported in red indicate that less than 90%

of results are achieving the standards and that action should be taken. If the report is in blue this indicates that the standard is within 5% of compliance and if the report is in black this indicates compliance with the standard. We have found this to be a very useful way of visually scanning the results of the SLA monitoring system for turnaround times.

Small sampling audits can be undertaken to audit other parts of the turnaround time, for example the time from the result being available to the time the clinician actually reads the result. It has been shown that the most significant factors in slowing turnaround times are poor arrangements for collecting specimens or returning results. The Audit Commission's report on pathology identified that these arrangements were often not managed by laboratories themselves, but the laboratory was initially blamed when things went wrong.[4]

Monitoring workload

Similar monitoring systems will need to be established to identify volume of tests for each clinical directorate. This is important to identify, even if no cross-charging for tests is carried out. Change in trends of activity should be identified since this may indicate either a change in service or a service development which has not previously been agreed. Monitoring systems which are used for cross-charging purposes should rely on data provided by the laboratory. Liaison with the finance department will be required if this process is to be established so that invoices can be cross-charged to clinical directorates.

In large laboratories there may be many contracts or SLAs to be monitored. It is therefore useful to develop a system of automatic reporting of all areas of activity. In our laboratory we have established an executive information system for this area. The system works by monitoring each area of activity, whether this is a SLA or an external contract. These areas then automatically feed into

Box 8.3: Monitoring of a service level agreement: chemical pathology and haematology turnaround times

% of test meeting SLA standard
Emergency service

Month Test	1	2	3	4	5	6	7	8	9	*Primary* *standard*
FBC	59	73	68	84	78	81	82	86	90	30 min
KCCT	25	57	61	57	62	59	57	82	96	30 min
C&E	78	73	87	79	82	88	79	73	86	30 min
Blood gases	98	95	100	100	96	98	96	96	100	30 min
										Secondary *standard*
FBC	75	83	80	89	88	88	91	91	96	45 min
KCCT	63	72	70	65	70	70	70	74	100	45 min
C&E	88	85	92	95	90	94	92	91	100	45 min
Blood gases	98	100	100	100	98	99	100	100	100	45 min

Priority service

	1	2	3	4	5	6	7	8	9	*Primary* *standard*
FBC	72	72	75	94	87	98	92	80	91	1 hour
KCCT	48	47	54	63	63	65	68	70	83	1 hour
C&E	90	90	96	99	96	97	98	95	95	2 hours
LFT	87	83	96	98	95	96	98	94	92	2 hours
										Secondary *standard*
FBC	83	82	92	99	97	95	96	92	95	2 hours
KCCT	84	92	88	79	92	97	85	92	96	2 hours
C&E	92	95	97	100	99	99	100	98	100	3 hours
LFT	91	87	98	100	99	97	100	97	100	3 hours

Routine service

	1	2	3	4	5	6	7	8	9	*Primary* *standard*
FBC	100	100	93	100	100	100	100	100	100	1 day
PV	99	100	98	100	100	99	100	100	100	1 day
KCCT	100	100	100	100	100	100	100	100	100	1 day
B_{12}	100	100	100	100	100	100	100	100	100	3 days
HbA1c	100	100	99	100	100	100	100	100	100	3 days
C&E	100	100	100	100	100	100	100	100	100	1 day
Cholesterol	99	99	100	100	99	99	100	100	100	1 day

summary reports so that an overall performance against contract is reported on a monthly basis as is shown in Box 8.4. For individual SLAs separate graphical displays are produced as part of this system so that we are able to monitor performance of each area separately.

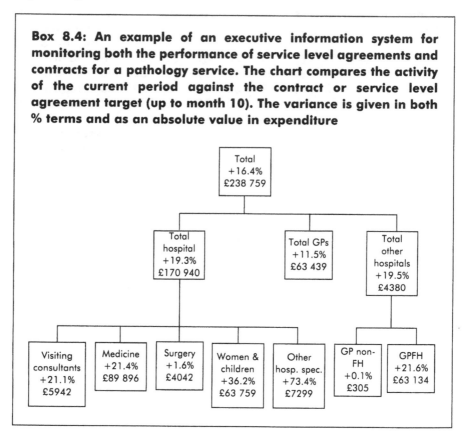

Box 8.4: An example of an executive information system for monitoring both the performance of service level agreements and contracts for a pathology service. The chart compares the activity of the current period against the contract or service level agreement target (up to month 10). The variance is given in both % terms and as an absolute value in expenditure

Establishing these monitoring systems and checking them for their accuracy is a time-consuming process. In the absence of this information, however, it is difficult to see how areas for improvement can be identified and service developments accommodated.

Monitoring laboratory requirements

Finally, users should receive feedback regarding compliance with the agreed standards of performance, for example completion of patient identification, compliance with protocols, etc. This type of monitoring is best achieved by sampling audits.

Conclusion

Introduction of SLAs has a potential benefit for laboratories in determining customer requirements, preparing business plans and agreeing developments. SLAs can also form the basis for identifying areas of underperformance and can therefore help to meet customer expectations. Both the financial performance of the laboratory and the quality of the service can be benchmarked against similar organisations. Financial performance can be compared by participating in the Clinical Benchmarking Company Study (Chapter 10). The quality of the service can also be benchmarked in the College of American Pathologists Q-Probes scheme (Chapter 6). It is clear that good, accurate and timely information systems need to be established as part of the process to ensure that standards set in SLAs are monitored and achieved.

Key point summary

- SLAs should be introduced primarily to facilitate quality improvements in the pathology service.

- SLAs should include agreement with users on the standards which they should achieve when using laboratory services.

- Detailed monitoring systems will need to be developed in parallel with the introduction of SLAs to ensure their successful implementation.

- Cross-charging for pathology services should only be introduced where clear benefit in financial control can be identified.

References

1 Galloway M, McHugh P, Shirley J and Ross I (1996) Developing service level agreements for pathology: Experience of the BAMM pathology group. *Clinician in Management.* 5: 6–8.

2 The Scottish Office (1992) *Specifications for Laboratory Services: guidelines for general managers.* Scottish Office Home and Health Department, Edinburgh.

3 KPMG Management Consulting (1992) *Laboratory Medicine Services in Scotland. Specification document.* KPMG, Edinburgh.

4 The Audit Commission (1993) *Critical Path. An analysis of the pathology services.* HMSO, London.

Further reading

Austin N and Dopson P (1997) *The Clinical Directorate.* Radcliffe Medical Press, Oxford. A good introduction to management, including a chapter on negotiating which is relevant to the introduction of SLAs.

Gilligan C and Lowe R (1995) *Marketing and Health Care Organisations.* Radcliffe Medical Press, Oxford. An introduction to marketing relevant to healthcare. This approach supports the introduction of SLAs.

9

Purchasing equipment

SUZANNE HARTELL

With tight budgets and little or no capital allocation for the procurement of pathology equipment, trusts are continually seeking innovative methods for funding, either to replace existing equipment which is no longer fully effective, or to acquire new, technologically advanced equipment. This chapter will discuss the various methods of procurement from leasing to private finance, and the pros and cons of each method. We will also explore the pathology market in general, to provide an overview of how the market is changing and how it is likely to develop in the future. The role of NHS Supplies will also be discussed, with details of the current structure and how the team can be contacted by pathologists. Finally we will touch on European Union procurement law and how this affects the procurement of pathology equipment.

Leasing in the NHS – an overview

With the recent clarification and relaxation of NHS private finance guidelines, more and more trusts are recognising that new financial initiatives allow opportunities to procure equipment, which may otherwise not be available to them. The inception of the government's private finance initiative (PFI) in November 1992 opened the NHS market to private sector funds, including leasing. Prior to this, leasing was regarded as unconventional finance, and could rarely compete with government funding of capital purchases. Hospital trusts previously acquired equipment using their capital budgets, rarely seeking external funding, or alternatively, they acquired equipment via reagent rental-type agreements whereby the cost of reagents was increased to offset the value of the equipment supplied.

HM Treasury produced guidance notes relating to leasing for government departments and the NHS in December 1992 and May 1993. Both these and the NHS Executive's own guidance notes stress that trusts should undertake a thorough analysis to determine value for money and risk transfer of any given financial options. In the case of a lease involving equipment whose capital is less than £1m, the NHS Executive guidelines state that the trust acquiring the equipment must demonstrate that the great majority of risk stays with the private sector. This test will be regarded as being satisfied if the lease counts as an operating lease under the SSAP21 accounting standard. Without the correct information, however, the decision whether to use leasing or other forms of finance can appear to be a complex process, particularly for non-financial managers wishing to prepare a business case.

NHS Supplies has experience of awarding leasing contracts for pathology equipment on behalf of trusts. It is the trust's director of finance, however, who has responsibility for authorising leasing contracts, and expert knowledge will be available from local trust finance departments to help guide you through funding regulations.

Definition of a lease

A lease is a commercial contract between a lessor (leasing company) and a lessee (NHS trust). The lessor retains ownership of the leased equipment, but the lessee has possession and use of it, in return for payment of specified rentals over a pre-determined period, which is typically three to five years. The lessor can be the supplier of the equipment, but equally may be a third-party finance company, who will purchase the equipment from the supplier and in turn, lease the asset to the trust.

The payment profile can be tailored to suit individual requirements. Payments can be tax-variable or tax-fixed over the lease period. The frequency of payments can typically be monthly, quarterly or annually, either in advance or in arrears. Payment of rentals forms the essence of a leasing contract, and timely payment must be ensured to avoid financial penalty or, in the worst situation, removal of the right to use the equipment. Product liability remains with the equipment manufacturer.

The operating lease

In an operating lease, the cost of the equipment, less a residual value (an estimation of the second-hand value of the asset at expiry of the lease), is spread over a pre-determined period which is always less than the useful, economic life of the asset. If the net present value (NPV) of the minimum total lease payments is less than 90% of the fair value (purchase price) of the asset, the lease qualifies as an operating lease (Box 9.1).

Box 9.1: Operating lease – coagulometer

	Discount factor	Repayments	NPV of repayments
Year 1	1	£3042.75	£3042.75
Year 2	0.9140	£3042.75	£2781.07
Year 3	0.8354	£3042.75	£2541.90
Year 4	0.7636	£3042.75	£2323.30
Year 5	0.6979	£3042.75	£2123.49
Year 6	0.6379	£3042.75	£1940.87
Year 7	0.5830	£3042.75	£1773.96
Totals		**£21 299.25**	**£16 527.35**

Total repayments	Purchase price	Risk transfer
£16 527.35	**£18 750.00**	**88.146%**

Financial details showing a discounted cash flow of an operating lease for a coagulometer. As can be seen from this example the net present value (NPV) of the repayments for the coagulometer over the period of the contract is 88.1%. Therefore this qualifies as an operating lease.

The contract is structured so that, for accounting purposes (and in accordance with SSAP21), it is considered to be off balance sheet and will count against revenue expenditure. Capital budgets are, therefore, not affected by the agreement and capital charges (at 6% of the asset current written down value) do not apply.

The finance lease

Any form of lease contract that does not qualify as an operating lease will, by definition, be a finance lease. Capital charges will therefore apply to the asset, and will attract a 6% cost against budget. As government exchequer funding is the cheapest form of finance, entering into a finance lease is not considered to be a cost-effective funding solution.

The reagent rental

Reagent rentals are often also known as managed service plans or operational management service contracts. In essence they are agreements whereby the trust will pay the equipment supplier one premium, which will include the rental of equipment, and costs of maintenance and all necessary reagents and consumables.

Since the premium is normally assessed against the given work-load in the laboratory, users entering into this type of contract must be able to define their workload fairly accurately and also what the likely increase will be over the contract period. Before entering into this type of contract it is important to define, as with any other lease, what the termination penalties would be at any given time, and also what effect a dramatically increasing or decreasing workload would have on the cost of the premium. Whenever possible, users should request a breakdown of the premium to define which elements pay for the rental of equip-ment, what proportion is for maintenance, and what proportion is for reagents and consumables.

This form of acquisition could, arguably, also be deemed as a finance lease and as such attract capital charging on the asset. Advice should be sought from colleagues in finance to ascertain the exact status of such agreements.

Private finance initiative (PFI)

Private sector funding is likely to become an increasingly important ingredient within pathology, either via NHS laboratories, undertaking research on behalf of specific suppliers or by a joint approach in the replacement of equipment.

Contracts awarded under the auspices of PFI will be complex in structure. It is important, however, to ensure, where possible, that all parts of the supply contract, such as equipment, reagent, supplies and maintenance, can still be clearly identified within the overall cost structure. This will allow such costs to be benchmarked against costs within other, more traditional types of contract, such as a simple purchase of equipment or operating lease contract. It should, of course, be borne in mind that a true PFI contract will be innovative, and as such, cost comparisons to show value for money must allow for other benefits to be accrued by the trust and the laboratory within the deal. Again, expert guidance from finance and supplies colleagues should form part of the process within a PFI scheme.

The contract

In order for a valid contract to exist between two parties, there must be an offer (such as a tendered offer to supply equipment by a supplier), acceptance of the offer as it stands and due consideration (payment in respect of the accepted offer). It is important to understand the implications of entering into a contract, whether it relates to pathology equipment of high value and strategic importance or indeed one box of test tubes of minimal value. The principles are the same for both items, in that an understanding of the terms within which business is being undertaken is of vital importance. Only the degree of possible risk involved will change between entering into each of the two contracts.

There are a number of standard sets of terms and conditions used within the NHS which are designed to minimise the risk to trusts when entering into contracts for the supply of equipment and consumables. Supplies colleagues will be able to advise on the appropriateness of these conditions.

Leasing – questions and answers

- *How long does a lease last and how are payments made?*
  The length of an operating lease must always be less than the anticipated useful, economic life of the equipment. Payments are made to the lessor, typically on a monthly, quarterly or per annum basis.

- *Does the equipment belong to the trust?*
  No, the lessor owns the equipment.

- *Can the trust upgrade equipment during the lease period?*
  Effectively European Union (EU) Supplies Directives (see p. 136) still apply when, for example, a new generation analyser is replacing an old one. Within EU law, which is incorporated within English law, it is not normally possible to 'swap out' analysers if there will be an extension to the contract term and/or an increase in costs.

- *What happens at the end of the lease?*
  Either the equipment is removed by the lessor or its agents and the trust has no further financial liabilities in respect of the equipment or, at the expiry of the lease, the trust can negotiate a secondary rental with the lessor based on the residual value of the equipment. This will allow the trust to maintain possession and use of the equipment for a further term.

- *Can the trust 'opt out' and return the equipment during the lease?*
  This is a possibility, however, the trust will normally be liable to pay a termination payment calculated by discounting all the outstanding rentals (typically at 5%). To avoid termination fees, it is important, when entering into a lease agreement, that users commit to a realistic term, dependent on local constraints and product life cycle.

- *Who is responsible for maintenance during the lease?*
  Maintenance and insurance responsibilities are treated in the same way as if the trust had purchased the equipment. The trust should ensure that the equipment is properly and regularly maintained.

Pathology equipment: the market

The total *in vitro* diagnostics market in the UK is estimated to be worth approximately £180m per annum shown in Figure 9.1. The split of reagents is estimated as shown in Figure 9.2.

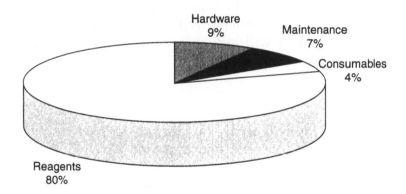

Figure 9.1 Total *in vitro* diagnostics market in the UK.

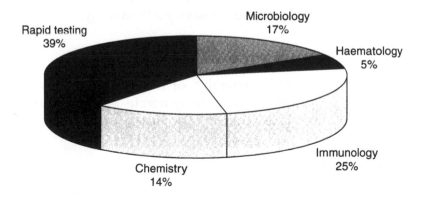

Figure 9.2 Split of reagents.

Structure and costs

Within pathology, it is normally possible to identify three main cost areas associated with pathology instruments, i.e. reagents, consumables and maintenance. The dominant costs will invariably be associated with the reagents. However, it is the total package which must be assessed when selecting instruments.

The market for mainline analysers is currently extremely competitive and prices offered reflect this competition. However, a number of factors will influence the total costs of the package offered. These are as follows.

Workload

The main factor will be the number of tests to be undertaken, normally assessed over a 12-month period. This will determine the revenue stream which the supplier can expect to receive, and will be the main department of pricing on equipment and reagents.

Mix of assays

This relates to the mix of tests to be undertaken. Each supplier is likely to have a number of tests which are not as profitable as others. This could be, for example, where the supplier markets a third-party supplier's reagent or where, to ensure accuracy and precision, it employs a more expensive methodology.

Strategic importance of site

A site that is high profile generally, or has an expertise within a specific area of testing, is likely to generate better pricing and could be used as a reference site by the successful contractor.

Length of contract

This tends not to influence pricing greatly from the closed system suppliers, where it is not possible to source third-party reagents. By the nature of their systems, the suppliers are guaranteed a revenue stream for the length of the operating lease or the economic life of the equipment. However, open system suppliers do offer good incentives for sites that will commit to the use of their reagents for a period of time, typically three to five years. These incentives can be given in a number of ways, including lower instrument prices, additional discounts of reagent kit price, inflation-proofed pricing and extended warranty periods.

General market

General market and product factors will also put pressure on pricing, such as the position of a supplier's instrument in its product life cycle.

As well as factors influencing the pricing submitted by suppliers, there are other factors which will affect the overall cost to the user. These are:

- reagent wastage
- sample loading
- calibration and control
- ease of use
- staffing.

The future market

The market for automated pathology instrumentation is moving extremely quickly. However, there is widespread belief that the following developments will happen over the next couple of years.

Supplier base reduction

The number of suppliers within the market will reduce. We have seen, over the past 18 months, several major acquisitions and mergers allowing suppliers to provide a wider configuration of instruments. There are likely to be financial benefits to a number of laboratories in having one supplier of these separate automated platforms, although it is difficult to gauge how significantly such developments will impact, especially on larger teaching hospital laboratories.

Equipment modulisation and workload consolidation

This involves having distinct modules which effectively bolt together to provide additional or rationalised capacity. This type of system will undoubtedly offer technical benefits, such as the provision of common sample handling and less hands-on use by laboratory staff. Standard centralised software will also be present.

Front end sampling

It is estimated that 70% of laboratory costs and 98% of the time to result are not associated with the analytical equipment. One of the main bottlenecks in the laboratory is the area of sample receipt. Technology is increasingly becoming available which allows for automation in the receipt, sorting, centrifuging and aliquoting of samples.

The role of NHS Supplies' purchasing division

The diagnostic medical equipment (DME) portfolio of NHS Supplies currently offers a limited, bespoke purchasing service to customers acquiring equipment of this nature. NHS Supplies acts as an agent of the trust in providing a project management-based purchasing service, which includes professional advice on commercial, technical and legal issues. There are also a number of contracts for the supply of pathology consumables available for use by trusts.

Key features of the DME portfolio within NHS Supplies

- purchasing service for major items of diagnostic medical equipment

- purchasing service for pathology and radiology consumables of strategic importance to the NHS

- national management of key, strategic suppliers

- tailored, limited purchasing service to meet the trust's specific requirements

- assistance and guidance in the preparation of business cases and specifications

- advice on alternative funding methods

- guidance in respect of legal, contractual and compliance obligations

- team of professional, national buyers

- commercial experience and expertise

- post-purchase support and advice.

Key benefits of working with NHS Supplies

- experience

- proven track record

- removal of duplication of effort

- concentration of core activities

- peace of mind about legislation and audit compliance

- cost-effectiveness and value for money can be demonstrated

- flexibility

- professional and independent advice

- increased negotiation power.

The DME portfolio structure

The DME portfolio ensures that all members of the team are equipped with a high level of both commercial and technical knowledge of the suppliers and products within specific market areas. A national approach to supply has been adopted by giving each buyer responsibility for a specific family of products and/or services. The structure is shown in Box 9.2.

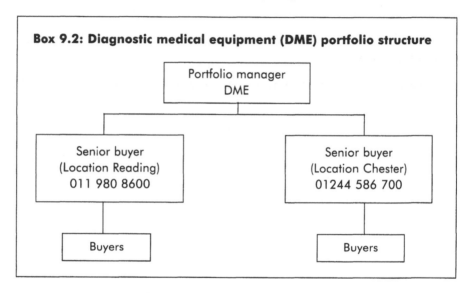

Box 9.2: Diagnostic medical equipment (DME) portfolio structure

European Union (EU) directives

In January 1973 Britain joined the European Economic Community (EEC) and as such became a signatory to the EEC Treaty of 1957 (The Treaty of Rome), which created the common market, permitting the free movement of goods, services, labour and capital within the community's boundaries.

The EU directives seek to ensure that public purchases achieve value for money, allowing competition from all member states, and ensuring compliance with good procurement practice. The directives provide a clear, procedural framework, which all purchasing and supply provisioning activities must remain within.

The directives' main provisions

- Contracts should be advertised through the *Official Journal of the European Communities (OJEC)*.

- Contracts should be put to competitive tendering.

- There should be a universally acceptable standard in specifications to promote wider competition.

- Evaluation criteria should be established early in the tendering procedure.

- Discrimination against foreign firms is prohibited.

Thresholds

The directives apply when the value of a contract or series of contracts exceeds £104 435 excluding VAT. This figure is amended by the Commission every two years, the next date being 1 January 2000.

It is expressly prohibited to split up a contract or contracts in order to take them below the threshold. In practice, the Commission considers that no question of splitting to evade the rules can arise if the contract value is calculated to include all the work necessary to make the service operational or provide the goods to the point of delivery.

Procedures

There are predominantly two procedures used in the procurement of equipment.

Open procedure
The open procedure means that any interested organisation is free to submit a tender. This procedure can be very useful in expanding purchasing horizons and broadening your potential supplier base. It can, however, be costly, as you are bound to provide an invitation to tender to all who request it and to consider all the tenders submitted. Additionally it can be resource intensive and a lengthy process.

Restricted procedure
Under the restricted procedure, only those suppliers invited may submit tenders, using the number of common, advertised criteria. The number of organisations invited must be sufficient to ensure genuine competition.

Conclusion

The key element in effective equipment management is planning. More and more laboratories are beginning to look at the long-term effect systems have on their environment and are establishing long-term relationships with strategic suppliers and other trusts to investigate and monitor the pathology market. It is important, when acquiring any piece of pathology equipment, that the user makes an informed choice which offers the best solution for the laboratory but also demonstrates value for money to us – the tax payer.

Key point summary

- Users should explore all viable means of funding to obtain best value for money.

- Effective contract management is a must.

- Expert advice is available through NHS Supplies and on-site finance departments.

- All contracts with a value above £104 435 must be advertised through the *Official Journal of the European Communities*.

10

Benchmarking laboratory performance

ROGER DYSON
HELEN ATKINSON

The 1997 White Paper[1] *The New NHS: modern, dependable* has amongst its key principles, '... a focus onto quality of care so that excellence is guaranteed to all patients ...', and '... to drive efficiency through a more rigorous approach to performance and by cutting bureaucracy so that every pound in the NHS is spent to maximise the care for patients ...'. The audit of quality is to go hand in hand with the audit of performance and in particular cost-effectiveness. The Government intend to benchmark the clinical performance of services with national reference data implemented through site inspections by the Commission for Health Improvement and implemented for cost effectiveness through the development of benchmarking.

For the lifetime of the 1997 Labour Government, therefore, benchmarking is here to stay and the objective of this chapter is to consider some of the issues around benchmarking laboratory performance and to illustrate one particular approach to benchmarking cost-effectiveness.

Issues in pathology laboratory benchmarking

In the limited scope of this chapter, the approach adopted is to pose the main challenges to benchmarking activity and to try to answer them.

In Clinical Pathology Accreditation pathology already has an ideal benchmarking system based on accreditation, why do more?
Clinical Pathology Accreditation (CPA) accredits laboratories on the basis of their achievement of at least two of the three key quality variables, namely input, process and outcome. CPA covers input and process but not outcome. CPA tackles the quality half of the benchmarking agenda but not the cost-effectiveness half. As these two initiatives are so clearly central to the new Government's policy, the need for something to parallel the achievements of CPA on the cost-effectiveness side are inescapable.

Measuring performance depends on an accurate measure of workload and this is difficult to achieve!
The first prerequisite is to ensure a balance of laboratory demand and supply. The demand on the laboratory comes as specimens from referring clinicians in the form of requests. Laboratory supply is the tests and investigations that are initiated in order to produce reports for the referring clinicians. Different requests require different volumes of testing and investigation, but even the same requests can be tested and investigated differently and as a result can lead to differences in cost. At the extreme end of the spectrum a microbiology department could generate almost an infinity of tests from a finite number of requests.

For this reason any measurement of pathology workload needs to balance supply and demand in calculating cost-effectiveness. It should balance requests with tests or sections, or blocks or slides in order to cross-check individual variations and this must be linked back to the type of work being undertaken. It is for this reason that laboratory supply must be measured on a like-for-like basis between different types of workload in order, yet again, to reconcile this with variations in the ratio of workload to requests. The principal failing of past and sometimes present workload measurement systems in pathology is the failure to measure and to balance both demand and supply.

Benchmarking can only really be successful if it can compare the costs of each item of workload.
The attempt to cost each item of laboratory work to a fraction of a penny has been a failed initiative for which the Audit Commission has been responsible in the past. Genuinely variable costs are only a tiny fraction of the total cost of an item of workload, although this proportion varies between departments. Whenever a formula is used for allocating the fixed costs it can cause the price of an individual item of work to vary considerably, and this is before one tackles the complication of a variable cost for the same item of work depending on which time of the day it is done. For this reason a pathology laboratory lends itself far more to an analysis based on average costing than on marginal costing, especially if that average is balanced in some way for greater or lower work-load complexity. The benchmarking together of laboratories of roughly equivalent size and clinical range reinforces the value of average over marginal analysis.

How can benchmarking work without site visits to prevent accidental or deliberate false data?
This is a legitimate question since none of the major cost-effective-ness benchmarking methodologies involves site visits. What can be done, however, is to clean the data in such a way that potential outliers can be followed up for data clarification. A good data cleaning system will always identify any meaningful accidental error, but deliberately false data are different. Core trust data are collected separately about trust revenue, staff, beds, clinical specialities, population, etc., and these data are linked to parameters of laboratory workload in order to check back with outliers. The same applies if the staffing does not balance with the salary costs, where similar parameters exist. This aspect of questionnaire management could be a chapter in its own right.

The Keele approach to laboratory benchmarking

At the time of writing this chapter the Keele University team has completed three years of laboratory benchmarking. After the first year this work was subcontracted by the Clinical Benchmarking Company (CBC Ltd) which is a company partly owned by the NHS Confederation. The pathology benchmarking team consists of nominees of the Royal College of Pathologists, the Association of Clinical Biochemists, the Institute of Biomedical Sciences and the British Association of Medical Managers together with a representative of CBC and two staff from Keele. Clinical and scientific representation dominates each of the pathology speciality teams and each team is responsible for the information collection proforma (the questionnaire) and the subsequent report. This team, known as the 'Expert Panel' has complete academic freedom and it in turn is advised by an annual feedback report from the participating trusts and their laboratory staff.

One of the great challenges of any benchmarking exercise is that those who are being benchmarked should feel that the process and the outcome are fair and should be able to influence the development of the process. As a consequence the Keele approach places great emphasis on a bottom-up rather than a top-down process of data collection, which can be illustrated in the simple diagram shown in Figure 10.1.

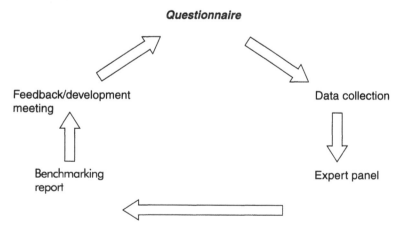

Figure 10.1 The Clinical Benchmarking Company – procedure for data collection.

Each year progress is made in improving and refining the process thanks to the help and enthusiasm of participating laboratories. For this a sense of ownership of the process is crucial. Each year virtually all the data are fed back to the participants in a report that is large and quite complex and requires it to be read and understood within the pathology departments themselves. The need for extensive data is crucial for fairness. Where a department is placed on a bar chart of performance is less important than why it is in a particular position, and the detailed data are meant to answer the question more effectively than the often erroneous assumptions of 'better' or 'worse'. Some departments have larger volumes or patterns of work; some departments are scattered whilst others are centralised; some have state-of-the-art equipment whilst others are struggling with older equipment and the same applies to information systems, etc.

Such a report requires an elaborate data collection exercise and this is always a challenge to overstretched departments. By collecting systematic data on a year-by-year basis, departments are increasingly able to develop software to collect data automatically and soon the opportunity of data collection by disk will be available.

With 78 laboratory participants in 1998 it was possible to undertake a meaningful clustering of laboratories by size and type in order to improve comparability. These clusters currently involve the traditional undergraduate teaching centres, the larger-than-average district general hospital (DGH), the smaller-than-average DGHs at or below 225 000 population with no major regional clinical specialities and the rest, which make up the largest cluster of mid-sized, non-teaching DGHs (clusters 1, A, C and B respectively – see Figure 10.2 for an example of how these clusters may be compared). There is scope for more precise clustering, particularly for specialist paediatric hospitals, and this process will become more sophisticated over time.

Some findings from the data

There is only space in this chapter to share three of the findings of the work as illustrations, the first of which is shown in Box 10.1.

The correlation between the volume of work and cost per request

We took the top and bottom ten volume sites as our two sample groups. We took their costs per request and found that the mean and the median of the two samples were consistently lower in the top ten volume sites. We tested to see if this outcome was statistically significant. We tested both parametrically using the unpaired one-tailed t-test assuming unequal variances and non-parametrically using the Mann–Whitney–Wilcoxon statistic. Both tests showed that there was enough evidence to suggest a difference between the two groups, i.e. the larger volume sites were producing a lower cost per request.

Box 10.1: The correlation between the volume of work and cost per request

	Clinical chemistry	Haematology	Microbiology
Top 10 mean	£3.84	£3.61	£4.75
Top 10 median	£3.50	£3.62	£4.50
Top 10 max.	£5.25	£4.05	£6.01
Top 10 min.	£2.67	£2.94	£3.71
Bottom 10 mean	£6.43	£5.47	£5.45
Bottom 10 median	£5.66	£4.78	£5.30
Bottom 10 max.	£12.85	£9.66	£6.50
Bottom 10 min.	£4.10	£3.49	£4.06
P-value (one-tailed t-test)	0.0053	0.0068	0.035

It is important to make the point that the message from these results is not that departments should be merged into larger factories, often off site. This is the simplistic solution that has bedevilled these comparisons in the past. Chemical pathology and haematology/blood transfusion require their bulk analysers to be on site for every hospital that admits acute surgical and medical patients around the clock. This is because hospital throughput and length of stay are much more dominant elements in cost-effectiveness than laboratory procedures. The availability of a service on site that is not dependent on delivering specimens away can have a crucial impact on turnover and length of stay, not to mention the clinical safety issues.

What the evidence shows is that for the smaller to medium-sized trusts with 24-hour acute medical and surgical admission there will be a higher cost per request, other things being equal, and that this is not a consequence of some inefficiency in organisation of staffing.

Are MLAs more cost-effective?

To see whether the ratio of MLAs to MLSOs had an impact on the cost per request we performed a simple linear regression analysis on the two sets of data. The results in each department showed a lack of relationship with R^2 as low as 0.09% in haematology.

In Figure 10.2 this conclusion holds only for the range of ratios between MLAs and MLSOs that are recorded in the chart. Nevertheless, those of us who talked about MLAs when they were introduced in 1989 as a potential for reducing costs in pathology have to admit that the evidence does not bear out this conclusion in any size of trust.

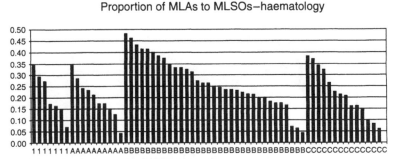

Proportion of MLAs to MLSOs—haematology

Figure 10.2 Are MLAs more cost-effective?

The correlation between the slide/request ratio and the cost per request in histopathology

As a final example we performed simple linear regression to look at the relationship between the number of slides per request and the total cost per request in histopathology (Figure 10.3). The correlation coefficient was significant at 82% and even when the three outliers were removed the correlation coefficient remained significant at 57%. We found enough evidence to suggest that cost per request rises with larger volumes of slides per request.

This is a new piece of work for 1999 and still remains to be tested more carefully over the next year or two before strong conclusions can be drawn. However, there is still a *prima facie* case to investigate, that the number of slides prepared may be one significant variable in influencing cost per request. There are still a lot of issues to address about stained and unstained slides, about how much material is on any one slide, and about what is done routinely under protocol for different types of biopsy and what is done only as the result of specific clinical request. Nevertheless, these findings are worthy of further investigation.

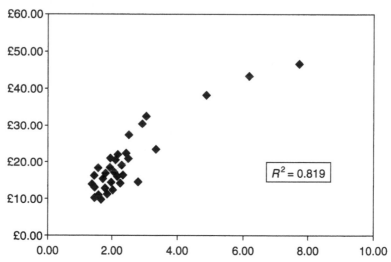

Figure 10.3 The correlation between the slide/request ratio and the cost per request in histopathology. Number of slides per request vs total cost per request.

Conclusion

The Keele pathology benchmarking review continues to grow as new laboratories join and the analysis of the 1997/98 data, which is now underway, will involve over one-third of all trust hospital laboratories in the UK. Whether this particular formula for benchmarking becomes the national standard in the way that CPA has become the standard for accreditation of clinical laboratories remains to be seen. Whatever the outcome, it is to be hoped that a participative system, allowing all laboratories to influence the process of benchmarking, will be sustained and that the search for fairness and transparency in benchmarking will continue.

Key point summary

- Benchmarking performance is a key part of government policy.

- The Keele approval for benchmarking laboratory performance is based on a participative approach including all users.

- The database for the benchmarking study has been developed to assess if organisational changes in pathology, e.g. the introduction of medical laboratory assistants, have been cost effective.

References

1 Secretary of State for Health (1997) *The New NHS: modern, dependable.* HMSO, London.

11

Changing working patterns

JANET SHIRLEY

Many laboratories are faced with changes in working patterns. These occur as a result of internal changes between departments in the same laboratory or because of service rearrangements between different hospitals due to laboratory mergers or whole trust mergers.

The aim of changing working patterns should be to improve the quality and cost-effectiveness of services, as well as addressing issues such as skills shortages, multidisciplinary working and flexibility. Since the publication of *The New NHS: modern, dependable*,[1] the emphasis is on co-operation rather than competition and this makes it easier to find new ways of working together. How changes are approached and managed, particularly in relation to staff concerns and perceptions, is crucial in successfully reorganising pathology services.

Internal laboratory reorganisations

Background

The drivers for internal laboratory reorganisations are many and varied. They can be divided into staffing problems, changes in technology, user requirements, and the drive for efficiency and cost-effectiveness as shown in Box 11.1.

There is a skills shortage in the UK at present and this means that it is becoming more difficult to recruit scientific staff at all levels. With the reducing levels of unemployment, staff costs are rising. Laboratories are being forced to look at changing skill mix, multiskilling and flexible working in order to recruit and retain staff and make the best use of their highly trained staff.

Box 11.1: Drivers for change in pathology

Staffing

  Scientific skills shortage
  Reducing unemployment
  Changes in training requirements

Technology

  Improved interaction between pathology services and their users
  – e-mail links to GP surgeries
  – computer terminals in wards
  Re-examination of the traditional boundaries between pathology disciplines
  – immunoassay
  – combined automated departments
  Automation in new areas
  – blood grouping
  – neural networks/telepathology
  – sample separation

User requirements

  Shift from secondary into primary care
  Near patient testing
  Increased day care, earlier discharges
  Acute admissions units, high technology medical interventions

Cost pressures

  Drive from purchasers for efficiency savings
  Market testing and the private finance initiative
  Changes in the configuration of acute trusts
  Lack of consultant expansion in pathology – problems with workload

---

Over the past ten years there have been massive changes in laboratory technology resulting from the introduction of fully automated analysers and fully integrated computer systems. This has driven the need to reconfigure departments along functional lines and to combine common laboratory functions such as specimen reception, data entry and sample separating.

User requirements 'have also' driven the change process. The introduction of admissions units, trauma teams and high technology medical interventions means that turnaround times for laboratory tests have become shorter. Also, results are required over the entire 24-hour period. GPs and patients want shorter turnaround times and extended laboratory access, and this affects the provision of laboratory services.

Along with all these changes there has been a drive for efficiency and cost-effectiveness in the provision of NHS services. This has been particularly acute in pathology because of the high cost of equipment and staffing. Many laboratories are being forced to look at alternatives for the provision of services when faced with budget cuts.

Internal laboratory reorganisations generally encompass two main areas:

- extending the routine working day or week

- changing departmental configurations.

For any type of change in working patterns the following areas require consideration:

- the implications of the proposed change

- managing the change process

- staff training and development.

The implications of the proposed change

Any alteration in the provision of laboratory services will have implications for configuration and staffing and there will be both pros and cons for the proposed change.

Geography of the department

When combining departments, such as the automated sections of haematology and chemical pathology, decide whether there is a suitable area within the laboratory complex to house the combined department. This also applies to combining common laboratory functions, such as specimen reception and data entry.

Resources required

New equipment or building works may be necessary in order to introduce the desired change and extra or different grades of staff may be required.

Management structures

The introduction of multidisciplinary working and merged departments necessitates a different management structure. Departments need to work closely together and can no longer be autonomous units.

Provision of a 24-hour service

There are several ways in which this can be achieved. Consider introducing new contracts for all staff or for new staff, replacing vacant posts with different types of grades of staff, persuading staff to change their hours and introducing annualised hours' schemes[2] as well as changing to full-shift systems.

Flexible staffing

This includes changing skill mix, multiskilling and flexible working hours. Job satisfaction, job enrichment versus job enlargement[3] and deskilling versus flexibility require consideration.

Staff concerns

Any change will result in changes to jobs and worries amongst individual staff about how the change will affect them personally. Service users may also be concerned about whether changes will influence the quality of the service offered to them and their patients.

Managing the change process

When introducing changes there are several essential steps to managing the process. These include planning, staff consultation and involvement, implementation, monitoring and management structures.[4] The introduction of multidisciplinary working and merging departments are the commonest areas of change within laboratories. This section will focus on these issues using the experience of combining specimen reception, data entry, sample separating, and the automated sections of haematology and chemical pathology.

Planning

It is essential to obtain agreement from the major stakeholders for any proposed change. Before starting to plan find out how the laboratory processes are currently carried out. We started with a specimen tracking project which identified that six different sections of the laboratory were, at the same time, involved in producing the results from one specimen taken from one patient. This also measured test turnaround times and gave us a base for monitoring service quality following implementation of the changes. Information was obtained on skill patterns (which jobs different grades carried out), activity and staffing levels (including skill mix), and productivity and cost analysis.

Following collection and analysis of the initial data, meetings should take place between senior staff in the departments affected by the proposed changes. An implementation plan, including the steps required to achieve the objectives, those responsible for actions and a timetable, should be drawn up and agreed.

Staff consultation and involvement

Following the planning of the change process, discussions should take place with staff in each department to identify how the objectives can best be achieved. This enables staff to be informed and involved and allows them to influence the changes. They will often point out snags that have not been identified or come up with innovative solutions to problems. The detailed planning of training and implementation is usually best left to the senior staff in each department or section. Where proposed changes affect the staff terms and conditions of service it is advisable to involve the staff unions in the consultation process. This reassures staff that management is not trying to drive through changes which are not in their best interests and is more likely to result in a successful outcome for all involved.

Implementation
In spite of careful planning, implementation is unlikely to occur without hitches. Regular review meetings should take place to monitor progress and identify problems. Flexibility is essential, as is the ability to modify objectives and timescales in the light of experience. Staff and users should be kept informed of progress.

Monitoring
The progress of the project should be monitored regularly with respect to timescales, achievement of objectives and costs. Following implementation, an audit should take place to identify whether objectives have been met. For example, we audited test turnaround times and unit costs post-implementation and showed that the two main objectives of improving service quality and reducing unit costs had been achieved. Assessment of staff satisfaction should also be carried out, particularly when changes have been made to job content or hours.

Management structures
Planning the management structure and getting it right is crucial in achieving change. When departments or parts of departments are combined, the classical management structure with a consultant head of department is difficult to maintain. Usually it becomes necessary to separate the line management of staff from the professional direction of a department. The consultant head of department should be responsible for the type and quality of the service, liaison with users, the development of business plans, the strategic direction and should play a central role in the management of laboratory staff. However, the day-to-day operational management of combined sections of the laboratory will be the responsibility of the senior scientific officer in that area.

Staff development and training

Many of the changes taking place in laboratories involve changes in skill mix and multiskilling of staff. These changes are occurring between clerical and MLA staff as well as between MLA and MLSO staff and have implications for staff training and development. Whenever planning change it is essential to identify training requirements and ensure that sufficient time and resources are devoted to these.

Changes in skill mix

Many of the jobs which were previously undertaken by MLSOs can now be performed by MLAs, following the introduction of automated specimen analysis and computerisation. Many data entry and monitoring processes are now performed by clerical, rather than laboratory staff. The introduction of a training programme for MLAs and supervision by appropriately qualified staff (Standard B3.2 for CPA[5]) means that these staff are properly monitored and reviewed, ensuring that service quality is maintained.

Box 11.2: Clinical Pathology Accreditation (CPA): training standards applicable to combined departments

B2   There are appropriate numbers of staff with the required training to ensure a satisfactory operation of service

Guidelines
1 All staff working in a multidisciplinary laboratory should be appropriately qualified and trained to CPSM standards (as set out in the logbook) in all disciplines in which they are required to work

B3   There is a documented line of responsibility for all staff

Guidelines
1 There should be evidence of the management structure, preferably using a schematic presentation. There should be a single documented head of department or director of service
2 There should be evidence that all unqualified staff are supervised by someone appropriately qualified

---

Multiskilling
This applies to MLSO, MLA and clerical staff many of whom now work across more than one laboratory department. Both CPA (see Box 11.2) and the Council for Professions Supplementary to Medicine (CPSM) recognise that this is a necessary training requirement and include the relevant accreditation and training standards. The CPSM now has a common core, common discipline-specific core and discipline-specific modules for the Medical Laboratory Technician's Board in haematology and hospital transfusion science, immunology and clinical chemistry.[6] This allows MLSOs to be trained in all these aspects of laboratory medicine and become truly multidisciplinary.

External laboratory reorganisations

Background

Many of the reasons for external laboratory reorganisations and co-operative working are similar to those driving internal laboratory reorganisation. Financial imperatives are common and purchasing programmes across trusts for laboratory equipment and reagents can generate large savings. These can be used to invest in new buildings and equipment which would be too expensive for a single trust. There are often specific local factors which make mergers an attractive option. For example, in West Surrey the centralisation of the Public Health Laboratories on one site left a trust without a microbiology laboratory and forced it to look elsewhere for this service. Threats from private laboratories have resulted in trusts collaborating in order to use scarce resources, such as equipment and staff, effectively and reduce their unit costs. Many acute trusts are merging in whole or in part, driven by the requirements of the task forces on junior doctors' hours and the new training programmes.

In the early years following the last government's NHS reforms it was very difficult for trusts to collaborate because of the competitive culture of the time. Many pathology departments were actively trying to gain contracts from neighbouring trusts, and in many case succeeding, and this created a great deal of distrust between laboratories. More recently the situation has changed and even before the publication of *The New NHS* many trusts had come to realise that collaboration is not a threat and can yield positive advantages. The will to work together to shape a new service is the most important factor in ensuring its success.

Principles behind external laboratory reorganisations

Many of the large external laboratory reorganisations, such as those in Lincolnshire, Leicester and the Leeds/Bradford partnership, started off in a small way with links between two laboratories in one or more pathology specialities. Following initial successes these have expanded to encompass all disciplines and other trusts and now involve pathology departments in up to five hospitals. Two main models have emerged, either a working co-operative or full merger. The differences between the two are mainly in respect of financial management and staff employment. The underlying principles for collaboration or mergers have been very similar, regardless of which model or which site is considered (see Box 11.3). The final configuration of services is also very similar as shown in Box 11.4.

Box 11.3: General principles behind external laboratory reorganisations

Background

> Cost pressures on purchasers
> Competition from other providers
> Need to maintain and improve service quality
> Successful initial collaboration with one or more speciality
> Problems in one or more speciality
> – cervical cytology
> – microbiology

To improve the quality, efficiency and effectiveness of the service leading to better patient care

> Utilise facilities and equipment more efficiently
> Increase the pool of expertise and level of consultant cover

continued

Increase the volume and range of specialist services, taking advantage of economies of scale

Reduce unit costs and maximise income

Improve training and development opportunities for staff

Improve recruitment and retention in a reducing labour market

Standards

Consultant advisory service across all sites

All acute pathology work from each hospital retained on site

Quality standards to be maintained or improved to meet user requirements

Merged directorates to function as a single pathology department

New directorate to meet the Royal College of Pathologists and CPA standards

Merged directorate to function as a single business unit

Box 11.4: Configuration of services following external laboratory reorganisations

- A core laboratory at each acute hospital site with haematology, blood transfusion, chemical pathology and acute microbiology

- A common IT platform with links between each site

- Single site cervical cytology, and in some cases histopathology processing

- Single sites for batch or specialist tests, although not necessarily the same site for all tests or all disciplines

- Common purchasing

- A standard staff policy

- A single financial mechanism

- A single management structure

Managing the change process

The principles behind managing the change process for external laboratory reorganisations are similar to those for managing internal changes within a single pathology department and should include planning, goal setting, staff consultation, timetabling and regular review of progress. There are, however, some specific considerations which must be taken into account in addition to the above, as set out in Box 11.5.

The consultation process should involve all stakeholders and particular attention should be given to concerns expressed by users of the service, particularly consultants in the individual trusts. The idea of a merger or collaboration should be discussed at each directorate before proposals are published and the proposals should contain a suggested management structure and a framework for consultation and moving the process forward.

Box 11.5: External laboratory reorganisations – managing the change

Consultation process to involve all stakeholders

    Users of the service – consultants, GPs, patients
    Staff at all sites
    Union representatives
    Personnel and finance staff
    Royal College of Pathologists
    Regional Postgraduate Dean

Project management

    Shadow board/project team
    Subgroups
    – each speciality
    – IT
    – personnel
    – finance

Merging the cultures

    Naming the new service
    Myths and stories
    Symbols
    Power structures
    Control systems
    Organisational structures

Modifications should be made in response to comments received, following which preferred options should be developed for service provision. These options should be presented to staff and users for further consultation.

Deciding on the configuration of services is best carried out by operational speciality subgroups. Each speciality should draw up a list of options, perform an option appraisal and identify problems. The views of CPA, the Royal College of Pathologists and the Regional Postgraduate Dean should be sought to ensure that training and accreditation requirements are met.

Merging two or more laboratory cultures may be difficult. It is important to decide on a name for the new service as soon as possible. People only begin to think in terms of the new organisation once it has a name; prior to this it is difficult to get away from 'them' and 'us'. Each department will have its own myths and stories, symbols and power structures. The organisational culture ('how we do things around here') and control systems (financial controls, IT, operational protocols and quality standards) may be very different and it is important to develop the new organisation and systems as quickly as possible.[7] It is essential to build a shared picture of the future, communicate the 'vision', overcome resistance and gain commitment from the key stakeholders.

When mergers occur the Transfer of Undertakings (Protection of Employment Regulations 1981) (TUPE) may apply and it is advisable to ask for legal advice. When TUPE does apply, the affected employees transfer automatically to the new employer on their existing terms and conditions of service. In some trust mergers, the individual trusts have continued to employ staff on prime site contracts so that no transfer of contracts occurs and TUPE does not apply.

Conclusion

Internal and external laboratory reorganisations are a common problem for pathologists and clinical directors. The most important factor in changing working patterns is to spend time on the staff consultation processes. Without the support of the staff it is impossible to manage these projects. Time spent in planning, identifying key stakeholders and selling the vision is time well spent and can prevent many problems. It is advisable to audit the quality of the service both before and after reorganisation in order to avoid accusations that the changes have resulted in a reduction in quality. Managing change successfully requires resources, in particular staff time, and investment in staff training and development.

Key point summary

- Internal laboratory reorganisations involve combining departments and using staff flexibly.

- External laboratory reorganisations involve collaborative working or full merger.

- It is essential to manage the change process.

- Staff development and training is a key issue.

- Staff and user consultation is essential.

- Merging the cultures is the key to success.

References

1 Secretary of State for Health (1997) *The New NHS: modern, dependable.* HMSO, London.

2 Shirley J and Fry I (1994) Extending the working day in the laboratory. *Bulletin of the Royal College of Pathologists.* **97**: 8–9.

3 Kopelman R (1985) Job redesign and productivity: a review of the evidence. *National Productivity Review.* 237–55.

4 Hansell D and Slater B (1995) *The Clinician's Management Handbook,* Chapter 8, *Project management,* pp. 126–41. WB Saunders Company Ltd, London.

5 Clinical Pathology Accreditation (UK) Ltd (1996) *Accreditation Handbook.* CPA, Sheffield.

6 Council for Professions Supplementary to Medicine, Medical Laboratory Technician's Board (1997) *The Board's Standards Logbook. Haematology and Hospital Transfusion Science, Immunology and Clinical Chemistry* (1e). CPSM, MLTB.

7 Austin N and Dopson S (1997) *The Clinical Directorate*, Chapter 4, *Managing change*, pp. 63–76. Radcliffe Medical Press, Oxford.

12

Health and safety

ELIZABETH GAMINARA

Ever since the industrial revolution, legislation has been enacted with a view to improving working conditions and Health and Safety (H&S) at work. Early laws tended to concentrate on specific workplaces and whilst in some instances this continues to be the case, current legislation tends to be more generally applicable to all places of work. There are few laws, therefore, which are directed solely at laboratory working and whilst some regulations are clearly specific, the others are more generally applicable and it is necessary to tease out the pertinent sections.

H&S in the laboratory is clearly of paramount importance and this, plus the loss of crown immunity in the late 1980s, makes it essential that clinical directors of pathology are aware of their responsibilities and incorporate a robust H&S programme into the routine of everyday working. The aim of this chapter therefore is to identify and summarise the most relevant aspects of the H&S laws and to provide a bibliography of the regulations, their interpretation and guides to their application. It clarifies the responsibilities of the clinical director and indeed all members of staff and in some instances describes practical ways in which H&S regulations can be implemented.

Background

The Health and Safety at Work Act 1974[1-5] is the basis of our current approach to H&S at work and failure to comply may constitute a criminal offence. It is an enabling act which means that additional regulations can be and are introduced at any time, without the need for full parliamentary approval. These regulations are published as Statutory Instruments (SI) and are legally enforceable. Recommendations on the implementation of SIs are issued by the Health and Safety Executive (HSE) in the form of an Approved Code of Practice (ACOP) or an Approved Method (AM). These codes of practice are not laws in themselves and failure to follow them may not constitute a criminal offence as long as the alternative practice adopted can be demonstrated to be equivalent. Numerous other codes of practice/guidelines are issued by government departments, expert committees and professional bodies but these have no official legal status. They may, however, represent good practice and in cases where negligence is alleged, deviation from such guidance may need to be defended in a court of law. An example of such guidance is *A Code of Practice for the Safe Use and Disposal of Sharps*[6] produced by the British Medical Association.

A comprehensive list of extant regulations, ACOPs and other publications can be obtained from the publishing branch of the HSE, HSE Books. Copies of individual regulations and guidelines on the list can be obtained from good bookshops, The Stationery Office or from HSE Books. The latter also publishes a wealth of HSE guidance leaflets, posters, videos, CD-roms and other training aids. The HSE provides an information service, a database of publications and a free subscription service *New Books News*, which provides a monthly update of new publications, statutory instruments and regulations. The relevant contact numbers and addresses for these outlets are shown in Box 12.1.

In most trusts there will be a H&S officer, and it is very likely that this officer, in conjunction with staff from the occupational health department, will already hold copies of some relevant publications. These staff members are well aquainted with the regulations and can provide invaluable assistance in negotiating the mass of information. They may also make a practical contribution by conducting in-house H&S inspections and audits and by highlighting areas of non-compliance or misinterpretation. Their expertise may also be harnessed to assist with staff education and training, by involvement in induction courses and ongoing programmes of more specifically directed training, for example manual handling or display screen usage.

Box 12.1: Health and safety resources

• Trust H&S officer

• Occupational health department

• The Stationery Office	The Stationery Office Bookshop
	123 Kingsway
	London
	WC2B 6PQ

Tel:	0171 430 1671
Enquiries:	0171 873 0011
Orders:	0171 873 9090

HMSO Publications
PO Box 276
London
SW8 5DT

• HSE	HSE Books
	PO Box 1999
	Sudbury
	Suffolk
	CO10 6FS

Tel:	01787 881165
Infoline:	0541 545500
HSELINE:	0171 323 7946/7

The regulations

In recent years, European legislation has had a significant impact on UK H&S law. As a result, a set of regulations were passed into UK law in 1992. These encompass many pre-existing regulations, update them and provide more detailed guidance on H&S relevant to the 1990s. Together with the other most relevant regulations, they are listed in Box 12.2.

There is significant overlap between the regulations, most notably in the requirements to undertake suitable and sufficient risk assessments, to remove risks where practicable but otherwise to take documented action which will minimise risk. Risk assessments should be performed using the most relevant and hence most exacting regulations and will therefore be deemed to comply with the less specific regulation and need not be repeated (e.g. a risk assessment undertaken to comply with COSHH regulations need not be repeated under the management of a H&S regulation). Another central premise is the requirement to provide staff with appropriate training, information and supervision and ensure that they are fully aware of their own individual responsibilities apropos H&S.

Box 12.2: The principle health and safety regulations

- The Management of Health and Safety at Work Regulations 1992

- Provision and Use of Work Equipment Regulations 1992 (PUWER)

- Manual Handling Regulations 1992

- Workplace Health, Safety and Welfare Regulations 1992

- Personal Protective Equipment at Work Regulations 1992 (PPE)

- Display Screen Equipment Regulations 1992

- Control of Substances Hazardous to Health Regulations 1994 (general, carcinogens and microbiological agents) (COSHH)

- The Reporting of Injuries, Diseases and Dangerous Occurrences Regulations 1995 (RIDDOR)

Brief summary of the regulations

The Management of Health and Safety at Work Regulations 1992[7-10]

This code of practice covers 17 regulations outlining the essential requirements of a H&S policy which should be integrated as a core activity of everyday working. It specifies clear lines of accountability and communication with evidence of a planned and organised H&S programme. There should be control, monitoring and review of the programme and this should be fully documented. One of the key activities to be undertaken is that of risk assessment and there is a requirement to 'identify significant risk', 'perform a suitable and sufficient risk assessment' of it, remove the risk if possible but if not, identify steps to be taken to reduce the risk, subsequently ensuring that these steps are actually taken. Where more than five people are employed, the risk assessments should be fully documented, the priorities should be set for action and the action subsequently undertaken. The regulations also cover the need to appoint a H&S officer and the need to have a H&S policy as well as policies to cover any potential major incidents. There is a requirement for access to competent external help and expertise, for example for purposes of health surveillance and for interaction with people external to the organisation on H&S issues. Finally, and very importantly, there is a requirement to involve employees in the process. They should have access to relevant information, should be given appropriate training and should be encouraged to understand their own role in H&S, taking an individual responsibility to keep up to date, avail themselves of training opportunities and generally incorporate safe working practice into their everyday activities.

Initially these requirements suggest the need for a large additional resource in terms of time, committee and paperwork. This need not, however, be the case, for as long as a department has a sensible management structure, with clear lines of accountability encompassing all staff groups, then H&S activities can be included on the agenda of the pathology directorate management team and cascaded down to all staff by way of individual departmental meetings. Documentation will follow automatically in the minutes of these meetings. Thought should be given to the position of the laboratory H&S committee in the management structure, one option being to report directly to the pathology directorate management team, making regular reports and bringing outstanding issues to pathology management team meetings. It is crucial that the pathology H&S programme interacts with that of the rest of the trust. This may be accomplished by agreeing formal representation on the trust H&S committee with the right to fill at least two and often more positions on the group. In practice, these are usually (but not always) filled by the pathology H&S officer and one of the consultant microbiologists, with other staff attending if they have a particular interest or expertise. In addition, the clinical director, who is accountable to the chief executive for H&S matters, can seek additional information, expertise or resource from outside pathology as appropriate.

Provision and Use of Work Equipment Regulations (PUWER)[11]

These regulations cover the use of equipment at work and include new, second-hand and leased equipment. They overlap significantly with other regulations, most importantly the management of H&S, in their requirement for risk assessment, appropriate training, instruction and supervision, and there is also some overlap with lighting at work and personal protective equipment, for example. Employers are reminded that the new equipment should comply with EC product directives, the most important of which is the machinery directive, the mark 'CE' on the equipment or the provision of an EC declaration of conformity, signifying compliance.

In general, equipment must be appropriate for the task in hand and should be designed for easy and safe working and maintenance. Where necessary, suitable guards should be used to protect against identified risks, control mechanisms should be in good working order, the environment should be adequate for safe use and where appropriate, hazard warning signs must be displayed.

Manual Handling Regulations[12-14]

Analysis of injuries at places of work (see RIDDOR) reveals that 34% of such injuries are related to manual handling issues. The problem is by no means restricted to 'industrial work' and the comparable figure for health services is 55%. The scale of the problem is recognised internationally and the regulations of 1992 are the result of a European directive which incorporates the modern ergonomic approach to removing or reducing the risk of manual handling injury. The regulations require employers to assess manual handling risks in the workplace, to remove them where possible but otherwise to minimise them and ensure that staff have the proper training and aids needed to prevent reasonably foreseeable injury. Problems may be prevented by improved design of loads and storage facilities and good organisation of work and rest periods. In most trusts the emphasis is on good nursing practice and patient lifting but there are significant manual handling risks in pathology, particularly for mortuary technicians but also generally, associated with the receipt, delivery and distribution of stores. Most occupational health departments will provide a manual handling training programme and this can be supported by the development of an in-house 'trainer' for day-to-day issues and ongoing training. Whilst all staff should be exposed to this at some time, it is probably only necessary to target certain groups on a regular basis (e.g. porters, mortuary technicians, some MLAs).

Workplace Health, Safety and Welfare Regulations 1992[15-21]

The matters covered by these regulations are very general and affect every employer and place of work. The approved code of practice covers a wide range of issues, including ventilation, temperature, lighting, cleanliness and waste. Details are given of minimum room size, minimum number of sanitation/wash facilities, organisation of traffic routes and flooring requirements. There are sections covering storage, windows and the need for vision panels in doors; there is reference to the provision of drinking water, rest and eating facilities, and the need for suitable facilities for pregnant/nursing mothers and for smokers. The document is of particular value for those departments designing new laboratories and close working with architects and works departments will ensure that most H&S features become an integral part of any new facility.

Personal Protective Equipment at Work Regulations 1992[22-23]

If there are risks/hazards in the workplace that cannot be removed but can be reduced by the use of protective equipment, then the latter should be provided to all employees, free of charge. The equipment should be effective and in working order and staff should be trained in its use, with documentation that this training has taken place (a simple signature confirming participation in a training module or explanation will suffice). Laboratory coats, which are mentioned briefly, along with gloves and eye shields, come into this category, whilst uniforms, which are not strictly protective, do not. Thought should be given to visitors to the laboratory and anyone staying longer than a few minutes should be given the appropriate protection, usually in the form of a white coat. Most laboratory staff are fully compliant with these regulations which are easily monitored by regular H&S audit inspections as well as ad hoc visits to the laboratory.

Display Screen Equipment Regulations 1992[24-25]

The principal hazards associated with the use of display screens are those leading to musculoskeletal problems, visual fatigue and stress. The risks are low; however, all the known health problems that may be associated with display screen work can be prevented by good design of the workplace or the job and by worker training and consultation. The guidance gives definition of a display screen user with illustrative examples. It describes how workstations should be assessed, giving sample checklists and describing minimum workstation requirements. It describes how work schedules and rest periods should be balanced and how eyesight tests and corrective appliances should be provided. Compliance is relatively straightforward with, for example, the training of a small team drawn from the relevant staff groups (clerical, data entry, MLAs, etc.) by the occupational health department with the help of the guidelines. This team can then assess workstations either as an ongoing process or as an annual 'blitz'. Findings can be reported to the H&S committee or the pathology management group, where any remedial actions required can be agreed.

Control of Substances Hazardous to Health Regulations 1994[26-28]

This legislation, updated in 1994, now covers, in addition to the control of hazardous substances in general, the control of carcinogenic substances and the control of biological agents. The latter regulation should be taken in conjunction with 'the categorisation of pathogens according to hazard and categories of containment'[29] and brings the handling of biological agents within the remit of the law. The duty of employers is not only to protect employees, but also, 'so far as is reasonably practicable', all other persons visiting the premises (e.g. junior doctors, cleaning staff and members of the emergency services). The three codes of practice include descriptions of hazardous substances, carcinogens and biological agents and describe the need to undertake suitable risk assessments. As with any risk assessment, the primary objective is to remove the risk, or otherwise to minimise and control exposure to the risk. There is a requirement for employers to maintain and monitor the control mechanisms put in place, to monitor exposure where it occurs and to keep records of the process. The records may take any format, as long as they are accessible and easily understood. They should be reviewed regularly. Examples are given of how exposure may be controlled particularly with respect to inhalation, ingestion and absorption. This section should be taken in conjunction with the reference document *Occupational Exposure Limits*.[30] This document is updated annually and provides lists of substances having either a minimum exposure limit (MEL) or occupational exposure standard (OES). It also describes methods of controlling and monitoring exposure, including the use of local exhaust ventilation. This is of particular relevance in histopathology departments with respect to ventilation of mortuaries, cut-up facilities, and the storage and distribution of formalin. Histopathology museums, with the potential for old, leaky pots, should not be forgotten, nor should controlled ventilation cabinets used in most laboratories. It is also of relevance to the control of the level of dust found in microbiology departments which make their own media.

The regulations state also that the employer should provide health surveillance where appropriate by suitably qualified staff in a suitable environment. In practical terms this usually means staff from the occupational health department who should maintain individual health records, institute a programme of immunisation where appropriate and investigate one-off episodes of significant ill health. Finally, employees should be given adequate information and training in order that they understand the risks and the controls and that they accept individual responsibility to comply with the regulations.

The sections devoted to carcinogenic substances and biological agents duplicate the general section in the main. There is, however, some more specific advice, particularly with reference to biological agents and this is directed at diagnostic and teaching laboratories as well as research and development establishments, including those using laboratory animals. It includes a classification of agents and describes minimum containment levels, giving a useful table of measures required to achieve each level. It outlines the requirement to maintain a list of employees exposed to group three and four agents, along with details of exposure, these records to be kept for ten, in some instances 40 years. There are also regulations relating to the use and storage of biological agents and the transport of biological agents/infected materials with the requirement to notify the HSE in certain situations.

From a practical point of view, it is essential that a systematic approach is taken to the implementation of the COSHH regulations and although this may be co-ordinated by the clinical director, it should probably be devolved via consultant heads of department, to each discipline under the direction of a senior member of laboratory staff. Implementation will be different for each laboratory but there is an extremely useful step-by-step guide available[31] in which a sequential framework of distinct stages in carrying out the assessments is suggested and which is of most relevance in the context of complex and serious risk. The point is well made that time and effort should not be wasted where risk is trivial.

The Reporting of Injuries, Diseases and Dangerous Occurrences Regulation 1995[32-34]

This regulation, which came into force on the 1 April 1996, replaces five sets of pre-existing regulations and stipulates that all significant work-related accidents, diseases and dangerous occurrences are reported. It applies to all work activities but not to all incidents. There is an abbreviated guide which describes how incidents may be recognised as 'significant', the main criterion being that the injury results in the loss of three or more working days. Dangerous occurrences which could have resulted in such an injury but did not, should also be reported and lists or examples are given. In addition, details are given of the more important work-related diseases, those relevant to pathology being hepatitis, tuberculosis and other infections. It also provides guidance in the completion of the standard report forms. The regulation is designed to identify areas of risk on which the HSE can focus in order to reduce injury, ill health and accidental loss.

Additional regulations and publications

In addition to the important H&S regulations detailed above there are other more general publications which may be of interest as shown in Box 12.3.[35-38]

Box 12.3: Other publications

- The Management of Occupational Health Services for Health Care Staff

- Surveillance of People Exposed to Health Risks at Work

- First Aid at Work

More specific guidance, directed at particular aspects of laboratory working, is also available and this, summarised in Box 12.4,[39-47] should be brought to the attention of all relevant staff groups.

Finally, there will be some laboratories undertaking more complex or specialised activities, in which case additional regulations will come into play. This may also be the case, albeit on a temporary basis, when laboratories are going through major operational or structural change. These publications are listed in Box 12.5[48-52] and the areas covered should be self-evident.

Box 12.4: Publications of relevance to laboratory working

- Safe Disposal of Clinical Waste

- Safety in Health Service Laboratories
  - Safe working and the prevention of infection in clinical laboratories
  - Safe working and the prevention of infection in the post-mortem room
  - Safe working and the prevention of infection in clinical laboratories – model rules for staff and visitors

- Safety at Autoclaves

- Principles of Good Laboratory Practice: notification of new substances regulations 1982

- The Storage of Flammable Liquids in Containers

- Introduction to Local Exhaust Ventilation

- Maintenance, Examination and Testing of Local Exhaust Ventilation

---

Box 12.5: Publications which may be of relevance

- The Radioactive Substances Act

- Approved Requirements and Test Methods for the Classification and Packaging of Dangerous Goods for Carriage

- A Guide to the Genetically Modified Organisms (Continued Use) Regulations

- Accommodation for Pathology Services

- Accommodation for Mortuary and Post-mortem Room

Conclusion

H&S is a rapidly changing area with new guidance being produced on a regular basis. For example, at the time of publication the NHS Executive had recently published initial guidance on the working time regulations.[53] Clinical directors need to be aware that there is a legal requirement for a robust H&S programme in all NHS trusts. Responsibility for this is delegated from the chief executive to the clinical director of pathology for implementation in the laboratory. Most laboratories give a high priority to H&S and will already be fulfilling many of the requirements to a greater or lesser extent. It is the task of the clinical director to manage and co-ordinate the H&S programme, ensuring that it is comprehensively applied and, through consultant heads of department and senior laboratory staff, is extended to every individual in the department in order that safe working practices become part of everyday working life.

Key point summary

- There is a legal requirement for clinical directors to implement a H&S programme throughout the laboratory.

- Guidance on the regulations and their implementation can be obtained from within the trust and from the HSE.

- It is not necessary to create a bureaucratic paperchase in order to implement a programme, rather, to build on whatever systems already exist in the organisation.

- The most important general regulations, plus some of those which are more specifically directed, are detailed and discussed.

- A comprehensive bibliography is provided for those seeking a more detailed knowledge of this area of legislation.

References

1   *The Health and Safety at Work, etc. Act* 1974. ISBN 010 54774 3. HMSO, London.

2   Health and Safety Executive (1992) *A Guide to the Health and Safety at Work, etc. Act* 1974. ISBN 0 7176 0441 1. HSE, Sudbury.

3   Health and Safety Executive (1994) *Essentials of Health and Safety at Work 1994.* HSE, Sudbury.

4   Health and Safety Executive (1992) *Health and Safety Starter Pack (Safety Representatives Version).* ISBN 0 7176 1352 6. HSE, Sudbury.

5   Health and Safety Executive (1996) *A Guide to the Health and Safety (Consultation with Employees) Regulations.* ISBN 0 7176 1234 1. HSE, Sudbury.

6   British Medical Association (1990) *A Code of Practice for the Safe Use and Disposal of Sharps.* BMA, London.

7   Health and Safety Executive (1992) *Management of Health and Safety at Work. Management of health and safety at work regulations 1992. Approved code of practice.* ISBN 0 7176 0412 8. HSE, Sudbury.

8   Health and Safety Executive (1997) *Successful Health and Safety Management.* ISBN 0 7176 1276 7. HSE, Sudbury.

9   Health and Safety Executive (1994) *Management of Health and Safety in the Health Services.* ISBN 0 7176 0844 1. HSE, Sudbury.

10 Health and Safety Executive (1997) *Managing Health and Safety: An open learning workbook for managers and trainers.* ISBN 0 7176 1153 1. HSE, Sudbury.

11 Health and Safety Executive (1992) *Work Equipment. Provision and use of work equipment regulations. Guidance on regulations.* ISBN 0 7176 0414 4. HSE, Sudbury.

12 Health and Safety Executive (1992) *Manual Handling: manual handling operations regulations. Guidance on regulations 1992.* ISBN 0 7176 0411 X. HSE, Sudbury.

13 Health and Safety Executive (1994) *Manual Handling: solutions you can handle*. ISBN 0 7176 0693 7. HSE, Sudbury.

14 Health and Safety Executive (1998) *Manual Handling of Loads in the Health Service*. ISBN 0 7176 1248 1. HSE, Sudbury.

15 Health and Safety Executive (1992) *Workplace Health, Safety and Welfare. Workplace (health, safety and welfare) regulations 1992. Approved code of practice and guidance*. ISBN 0 7176 0413 6. HSE, Sudbury.

16 Health and Safety Executive (1997) *Workplace Health, Safety and Welfare Regulations: a short guide*. ISBN 0 7176 1328 3. HSE, Sudbury.

17 Health and Safety Executive (1997) *Lighting at Work*. ISBN 0 7176 1232 5. HSE, Sudbury.

18 Health and Safety Executive (1997) *Seating at Work*. ISBN 0 7176 1231 7. HSE, Sudbury.

19 Health and Safety Executive (1993) *Electricity at Work: safe working practices*. ISBN 0 7176 0442 X. HSE, Sudbury.

20 Health and Safety Executive (1995) *Stress at Work: a guide for employers*. ISBN 0 7176 0733 X. HSE, Sudbury.

21 Health and Safety Executive (1996) *Slips and Trips: guidance for employers on identifying hazards and controlling risks*. ISBN 0 7176 1145 0. HSE, Sudbury.

22 Health and Safety Executive (1992) *Personal Protective Equipment at Work. Personal protective equipment at work regulations 1992. Guidance on regulations*. ISBN 0 07176 0415 2. HSE, Sudbury.

23 Health and Safety Executive (1992) *A Short Guide to the Personal Protective Equipment at Work Regulations 1992*. ISBN 0 7176 0889 1. HSE, Sudbury.

24 Health and Safety Executive (1992) *Display Screen Equipment Work. Health and safety (display screen equipment) regulations 1992. Guidance on the regulations*. ISBN 0 7176 0410 1. HSE, Sudbury.

25 Health and Safety Executive (1994) *VDUs: an easy guide to the regulations.* ISBN 0 7176 0735 6. HSE, Sudbury.

26 Statutory Instrument No. 3246 (1994) *The Control of Substances Hazardous to Health Regulations.* HMSO, London.

27 Health and Safety Executive (1995) *General COSHH ACOP and Carcinogens ACOP and Biological Agents ACOP. Control of substances hazardous to health regulations 1994.* HSE, Sudbury.

28 Health and Safety Executive (1989) *COSHH: an open learning course.* ISBN 0 7176 0850 6. HSE, Sudbury.

29 Advisory Committee on Dangerous Pathogens (1995) *Categorisation of Pathogens According to Hazard and Categories of Containment* (4e) HSE, Sudbury.

30 EH 40/96 (1996) *Occupational Exposure Limits.* ISBN 0 7176 1021 7. HSE, Sudbury.

31 Health and Safety Executive (1993) *A Step by Step Guide to COSHH Assessments.* ISBN 0 11 886379 7. HSE, Sudbury.

32 Statutory Instrument (1985) No. 2023 (1995) *The Reporting of Injuries Diseases and Dangerous Occurrences Regulations.* ISBN 0 11 058023 0. HMSO, London.

33 Health and Safety Executive (1995) *A Guide to the Reporting of Injuries, Diseases and Dangerous Occurrences Regulations 1985.* ISBN 0 7176 0432 2. HSE, Sudbury.

34 Health and Safety Executive (1995) *Everyone's Guide to RIDDOR 95.* ISBN 0 7176 1077 2. HSE, Sudbury.

35 Tivey DJ (1993) *The Management of Occupational Health Services for Healthcare Staff.* ISBN 0 11 882127 X. HMSO, London.

36 Health and Safety Executive (1990) *Surveillance of People Exposed to Health Risks at Work.* ISBN 0 7176 0525 6. HSE, Sudbury.

37 Health and Safety Executive (1997) *First Aid at Work. The health and safety first-aid at work regulations 1981. Approved code of practice and guidance.* ISBN 0 7176 1050 0. HSE, Sudbury.

38 Health and Safety Executive (1997) *Violence and Aggression to Staff in the Health Services: guidance on assessment and management.* ISBN 0 7176 1466 2. HSE, Sudbury.

39 NHS Executive Health Guidance Note (1995) *Safe Disposal of Clinical Waste Whole Hospital Policy Guidance.* HMSO, London.

40 Health Services Advisory Committee (1995) *Safety in Health Service Laboratories: safe working and the prevention of infection in clinical laboratories.* HMSO, London.

41 Health Services Advisory Committee (1991) *Safety in Health Service Laboratories: safe working and the prevention of infection in the mortuary and post-mortem room.* HMSO, London.

42 Health Services Advisory Committee (1991) *Safety in Health Service Laboratories: safe working and the prevention of infection in clinical laboratories: model rules for staff and visitors.* HMSO, London.

43 Health and Safety Executive Guidance Notes PM73 (2e) (1998) *Safety at Autoclaves.* ISBN 0 7176 1534 0. HSE, Sudbury.

44 Principles of good laboratory practice (1982) *Notification of New Substances Regulations 1982. In support of SI 1982,* No. 1496. ISBN 0 11 883658 7. HMSO, London.

45 Health and Safety Executive (1998) *The Storage of Flammable Liquids in Containers. Revised.* ISBN 0 7176 1471 9. HSE, Sudbury.

46 Health and Safety Executive (1993) *Introduction to Local Exhaust Ventilation. 1993.* ISBN 0 7176 1001 2. HSE, Sudbury.

47 HS (G) 54 (1990) *The Maintenance, Examination and Testing of Local Exhaust Ventilation.* ISBN 0 11 885438 0. HSE, Sudbury.

48 *The Radioactive Substances Act 1993.* CH 12. ISBN 010 5412937. HMSO, London.

49 Health and Safety Executive (1996) *The Carriage of Dangerous Goods Explained. Part 1. Guidance for consignors or dangerous goods by road and rail (classification, packaging, labelling and provision of information).* ISBN 0 7176 1255 4. HSE, Sudbury.

50 Health and Safety Executive (1996) *A Guide to the Genetically Modified Organisms (Contained Use) Regulations 1992 as amended in 1996.* ISBN 0 7176 1186 8. HSE, Sudbury.

51 NHS Estates (1991) *Health Building Note 15. Accommodation for pathology services.* HMSO, London.

52 NHS Estates (1990) *Health Building Note 20. Accommodation for ortuary and post-mortem room.* HMSO, London.

53 HSC 1998/160 (1998) *The Working Time Regulations: NHS Executive guidance.* NHS Executive, London.

Appendix: Useful addresses

Association of Clinical Pathologists
189 Dyke Road
Hove
East Sussex BN3 1TL

Tel: 01273 775700
Fax: 01273 773303
E-mail: *info@pathologists.org.uk*
http://www.pathologists.org.uk

British Association of Medical Managers
3rd Floor
Petersgate House
St Petersgate
Stockport SK1 1HE

Tel: 0161 474 1141
Fax: 0161 474 7167
E-mail: *bamm@premier.co.uk*

Central Consultants and Specialists Committee
British Medical Association
BMA House
Tavistock Square
London WC1H 9JP

Tel: 0171 383 6059
Fax: 0171 383 6766
http://www.bma.org.uk

Clinical Benchmarking Company
25 Christopher Street
London EC2A 2BS

Tel: 0171 422 0295
Fax: 0171 422 0234

Clinical Management Unit
Centre of Health Planning and Management
Suite 1.18
Darwin Building
Keele University
Staffordshire ST5 5SR

Tel: 01782 583439
Fax: 01782 717732

Clinical Pathology Accreditation (UK) Ltd
45 Rutland Park
Botanical Gardens
Sheffield S10 2PB

Tel: 0114 268 6151
Fax: 0114 268 6251
E-mail: *office@cpa-uk.co.uk*

Health and Safety Executive Books
PO Box 1999
Sudbury
Suffolk CO10 6FS

Tel: 01787 881165
Infoline: 0541 545500
HSELine: 0171 323 7946/7
Further health and safety information can also be found at
http://www.open.gov.uk

Institute of Biomedical Science
12 Coldbath Square
London EC1R 5HL

Tel: 0171 636 8192
Fax: 0171 436 4946
http://www.ibms.org

NHS Supplies
80 Lightfoot Street
Chester CH2 3AD

Tel: 01244 586700
               01244 586760

Q-Probes
College of American Pathologists
325 Waukegan Road
Northfield
Illinois 60093-2750
USA

Tel: 001 847 832 7000 (from the UK)
Fax: 001 847 832 8168 (from the UK)
http://www.cap.org

Royal College of Pathologists
2 Carlton House Terrace
London SW1Y 5AF

Tel: 0171 930 5861
Fax: 0171 321 0523
http://www.rcpath.org

Standing Committee on Postgraduate Medical & Dental Education
1 Park Square West
London NW1 4LJ

Tel: 0171 935 3916
Fax: 0171 935 8601
E-mail: *secretary@scopme.org.uk*
http://www.scopme.org.uk

Index

Milton Keynes UK
Ingram Content Group UK Ltd.
UKHW031149141024
449569UK00024B/942